# Refractory Celiac Disease

Georgia Malamut • Nadine Cerf-Bensussan

Editors

# Refractory Celiac Disease

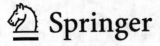 Springer

*Editors*
Georgia Malamut
Department of Gastroenterology
AP-HP. Centre-Université de Paris
Hôpital Cochin
Paris, France

Nadine Cerf-Bensussan
Laboratory of Intestinal Immunity
Université de Paris, INSERM UMR 1163
and Imagine Institute
Paris, France

ISBN 978-3-030-90144-8      ISBN 978-3-030-90142-4   (eBook)
https://doi.org/10.1007/978-3-030-90142-4

This Springer imprint is published by the registered company Springer Nature Switzerland AG
The registered company address is: Gewerbestrasse 11, 6330 Cham, Switzerland

# Contents

# Introduction

**Georgia Malamut and Nadine Cerf-Bensussan**

Coeliac disease (CD) has customarily a benign outcome after gluten-free diet with symptoms that resolve within a few weeks while normal epithelial architecture is recovered within one to two years (see text by S Varma, S Krishnareddy). Yet, iterative follow-up of biopsies has revealed that histological recovery is delayed in some patients. Notably one population-based study led in 7648 celiac patients in Sweden showed persistent villous atrophy in 43% cases among individuals biopsied one to two years and two to five years after diagnosis [1]. Persistent symptoms and villous atrophy are mainly due to bad observance to a gluten free diet (GFD) [2]. Nevertheless, a small group of CD patients may be primarily or secondary resistant to a GFD due to an authentic refractory celiac disease (RCD). Diagnosis of this condition is made after exclusion of other intestinal diseases with villous atrophy (see text by Huloel and J. Murray). Drug induced enteropathy such as olmesartan-induced enteropathy can mimic refractory coeliac disease but is usually easy to recognize based on anamnesis [3, 4]. In contrast, enteropathy associated with primary hypogammaglobulinemia and autoimmune enteropathy represent challenging differential diagnoses given the overlap between clinical presentation and autoimmune background [5, 6]. In the latter entities, genetic investigation may provide clues for personalized therapy [7].

G. Malamut (✉)
Department of Gastroenterology, AP-HP. Centre-Université de Paris Hôpital Cochin, Paris, France

Université de Paris, INSERM UMR 1163 and Imagine Institute, Laboratory of Intestinal Immunity, Paris, France
e-mail: georgia.malamut@aphp.fr

N. Cerf-Bensussan
Laboratory of Intestinal Immunity, Université de Paris, INSERM UMR 1163 and Imagine Institute, Paris, France
e-mail: nadine.cerf-bensussan@inserm.fr

Authentic refractory coeliac disease (RCD) refers to persistence of malnutrition and intestinal villous atrophy for more than one to two years despite strict gluten-free diet in coeliac patients having initially serum detectable coeliac antibodies and coeliac susceptibility haplotype HLA-DQ2 or -DQ8. Ascertaining diagnosis remains difficult and impacts treatment and follow-up. RCD has been subdivided into two subgroups according to the normal (RCDI) or abnormal phenotype of intraepithelial lymphocytes (IEL) (RCDII). RCDII is considered as a low-grade intraepithelial lymphoma and has a poor prognosis due to gastrointestinal and extra-intestinal dissemination of the abnormal IELs, and high risk of overt lymphoma [8]. Exact incidence and prevalence of either type of RCD remains unknown even if estimations can be performed on the basis of published series (see in this book K. Lundin, K. Kaukinen). One obstacle impairing true estimation of RCD frequency is the difficulty to ascertain diagnosis. Indeed, no specific criterium allows distinguishing RCDI from active coeliac disease, except for the demonstration of strict adherence to gluten free diet. Tests detecting gluten immunogenic peptides in stool or urine have been developed in order to complete dietitian survey and coeliac serology and to confirm good observance to gluten free diet (see in this book S Varma, S Krishnareddy). Diagnosis of RCDII is straighter. First, clinical presentation is noisy with ulcerative jejunitis and, as a consequence, protein loss enteropathy in about 70% of patients at diagnosis [8] (see text by HA Penny, C Zammat, DS Sanders). Second, strict criteria exist based on combined immunohistochemistry, flow cytometry and molecular analyses [8]. These diagnostic tools are notably useful to differentiate RCDII from so-called indolent intestinal T cell lymphoproliferations [9, 10] (see in this book D. Cazal-Hatem, G. Malamutand, L. Lhermitte, N. Cerf-Bensusan, S. Cording). Differential diagnosis between RCDI and II is indispensable as their prognosis, treatment and outcome differ radically. RCDI has a favourable prognosis close to that of uncomplicated coeliac disease. Its treatment relies on open capsule budesonide and immunosuppressive drugs [8]. On the contrary, prognosis of RCDII is poor mainly due to malnutrition and high risk of overt lymphoma called Enteropathy Associated T cell Lymphoma (see text by D. Sibon & O. Hermine). Prognostic scores have been established in order to predict RCD outcome (See text by A Schiepatti & F Biagi). There is no evidence or indication to support the use immunosuppressive drugs such as cyclosporine, azathioprine and anti-TNF-alpha antibodies in RCDII due to lack of efficacy and risk of hastening transformation into EATL [11]. Open capsule budesonide appears as the first line treatment in RCDII: it is generally efficacious to obtain villous recovery and to decrease the number of abnormal lymphocytes while having much lower iatrogenic effects than more aggressive drugs such as cladribine and fludarabine, two purine analogs that are used in RCDII refractory to steroids particularly in association with autologous stem cell transplantation. Recent advances in RCDII pathogenesis have opened the path to targeted therapy (see text by S. Cording, S. Berrabah, G. L. Lhermitte, Malamut, N. Cerf-Bensussan). A clinical trial using a blocking anti-IL-15 led two years a ago showed disappointing efficacy. Following identification of recurrent somatic mutations in the JAK1/STAT3 pathway in RCDII lymphocytes, JAK inhibitors are currently tested in a Phase 2 clinical trial with the goal to inhibit the growth and activation of malignant cells that is driven by the inflammatory cytokines upregulated in the celiac intestine (see text by k G. Bouma and T. Dieckman). Besides specific therapy, prognostic scores demonstrated the needs to restore serum albumin and hemoglobin levels, in order to improve long term survival.

We thank the authors of the present book, who are all specialized in refractory celiac disease and have accepted to share their expertise in order to provide an exhaustive presentation of epidemiological, diagnostic, pathogenic and therapeutic aspects of refractory coeliac disease.

# References

1. Lebwohl B, Murray JA, Rubio-Tapia A, et al. Predictors of persistent villous atrophy in coeliac disease: a population-based study. Aliment Pharmacol Ther. 2014;39:488–95.
2. Vahedi K, Mascart F, Mary JY, et al. Reliability of antitransglutaminase antibodies as predictors of gluten-free diet compliance in adult celiac disease. Am J Gastroenterol. 2003;98:1079–87.
3. Rubio-Tapia A, Herman M, Ludvigsson J, et al. Severe spruelike enteropathy associated with olmesartan. Mayo Clin Proc. 2012;87(8):732–8.
4. Scialom S, Malamut G, Meresse B, et al. Gastrointestinal disorder associated with olmesartan mimics autoimmune enteropathy. PLoS One. 2015;10:e0125024.
5. Malamut G, Verkarre V, Suarez F, et al. The enteropathy associated with common variable immunodeficiency: the delineated frontiers with celiac disease. Am J Gastroenterol. 2010;105:2262–75.
6. Akram S, Murray JA, Pardi DS, et al. Adult autoimmune enteropathy: Mayo Clinic Rochester experience. Clin Gastroenterol Hepatol. 2007;5:1282–90.
7. Parlato M, Charbit-Henrion F, Abi Nader E, et al. Efficacy of ruxolitinib therapy in a patient with severe enterocolitis associated with a STAT3 gain-of-function mutation. Gastroenterology. 2019;156:1206–10.c1.
8. Malamut G, Afchain P, Verkarre V, et al. Presentation and long-term follow-up of refractory celiac disease: comparison of type I with type II. Gastroenterology. 2009;136:81–90.
9. Malamut G, Meresse B, Verkarre V, et al. Large granular lymphocytic leukemia: a treatable cause of refractory celiac disease. Gastroenterology. 2012;143(6):1470–2.
10. Malamut G, Meresse B, Kaltenbach S, et al. Small intestinal CD4+ T-cell lymphoma is a heterogenous entity with common pathology features. Clin Gastroenterol Hepatol. 2014;12(4):599–608.
11. Tack GJ, Van Asseldonk DP, Van Wanrooij RLJ, et al. Tioguanine in the treatment of refractory coeliac disease - a single centre experience. Aliment Pharmacol Ther. 2012;36(3):274–81.

# Uncomplicated Celiac Disease

**Sanskriti Varma and Suneeta Krishnareddy**

## Introduction

Celiac disease is a chronic, autoimmune systemic disorder triggered by the ingestion of gluten, a protein found in foods such as wheat, rye, and barley. It is also known as gluten-sensitive enteropathy, non-tropical sprue, celiac sprue, and gluten-induced enteropathy. The disease process mainly affects the small intestine, amongst those with a genetic predisposition of acquiring the disease, nuanced by dietary and environmental factors [1]. Celiac disease leads to chronic inflammation of the small intestinal mucosa, which leads to atrophy of the intestinal villi and subsequent malabsorption. Celiac disease can develop and produce clinical manifestations at any age.

Greek physician and medical writer Aretaeus of Cappadocia was the first to describe celiac disease, referred to as "the Coeliac Affection" in Rome around 50 AD. Celiac disease was then re-described by Samuel Gee in the 1800s. He referred to the appearance of stools, onset of the condition, muscular weakness, abdominal distention, and chronic course of the disease, also noting that diet played a big role in disease. The cause was overall unexplained until Dutch pediatrician Willem K Dicke described an associated between the consumption of bread and cereals in children with remitting and relapsing diarrhea [2, 3]. Future supporting observations were noted during the periods of food shortage in World War II, when patients had improvement in symptomatology once bread was replaced by

S. Varma (✉)
Department of Internal Medicine, NewYork-Presbyterian, Columbia University Irving
Medical Center, New York, NY, USA

S. Krishnareddy
Division of Digestive and Liver Diseases, NewYork-Presbyterian, Columbia University Irving
Medical Center, New York, NY, USA
e-mail: sk3222@cumc.columbia.edu

© Springer Nature Switzerland AG 2022
G. Malamut, N. Cerf-Bensussan (eds.), *Refractory Celiac Disease*,
https://doi.org/10.1007/978-3-030-90142-4_2

non-cereal-containing foods [2]. Shortly after, extensive experimentation found that wheat, barley, rye, and oats triggered malabsorption and that these agents were present in gluten (the alcohol-soluble fraction of wheat protein) [4, 5].

## Epidemiology

Celiac disease occurs largely in patients of European ancestry. It is also seen among those of Middle Eastern, Indian, South American, and North African descent. It is rarely seen in Asians. Celiac disease affects about 1% of the United States population [6]. The worldwide prevalence of celiac disease is 1.4% based on blood tests and 0.7% based on biopsy results. The prevalence of celiac disease is 0.4% in South America, 0.5% in Africa, 0.5% in North America, 0.6% in Asia, and 0.8% in Europe and Australia [6]. While celiac disease may present in both children and adults, the average age at diagnosis worldwide is 48 years in men and 45 years in women [7]. Furthermore, the prevalence is estimated to be 1.5 to 2 times higher among females as compared to males [8]. Overall, prevalence of disease varies with sex, age, and geographic location.

## Pathogenesis and Risk Factors

The pathogenesis and risk factors of celiac disease are dependent upon the complex interaction between genetics, reaction to gluten, and other environmental factors.

Dietary gluten is a key exposure that plays into the development of celiac disease; those who are not exposed to gluten do no develop celiac disease. This dietary dependence sets celiac disease apart from other autoimmune disorders. Gluten is pervasive in the Western diet. It is a type of protein, which encompasses both gliadins (monomeric proteins) and glutenins (polymeric aggregated proteins) [9, 10]. Gluten and its components (glutenin and gliadin) are rich in alcohol soluble proline and glutamine peptides; these peptides are poorly digested in the human gastrointestinal tract because they resist degradation by luminal and brush border endopeptidases [11]. Once in the digestive tract, gluten is incompletely digested into gliadin fragments that gain entry through the epithelial barrier of the intestinal mucosa due to increased mucosal permeability [11]. Thereafter, the enzyme tissue transglutaminase (an ubiquitous intracellular enzyme) deamidates gliadin and renders it a more immunogenic molecule [12]. The latter is a significant step in the pathogenesis of celiac disease.

Gluten peptides have been implicated as triggers of innate responses in intestinal epithelial and mononuclear cells [13]. Innate responses to gluten are involved in the initial immune response, and are thought to further trigger the gliadin-specific adaptive T-cell response in genetically predisposed individuals. There is an increased production of cytokines, particularly IL-15, proliferated by enterocytes, macrophages, and dendritic cells [14]. This leads to differentiation of intraepithelial lymphocytes into cytotoxic CD8+ T cells that express the natural killer cell marker NK-G2D [15]. Ultimately, this inflammatory cascade leads to damage of the intestinal mucosa, manifesting as the classic histologic features of villous atrophy and crypt hyperplasia (characteristic histologic findings of celiac).

The adaptive immune response to gliadin involves antigen-presenting cells (macrophages, dendritic cells, B cells), which express the HLA class II DQ2 and/or DQ8 molecules on their surfaces and uptake and display gliadin proteins. These antigen-presenting cells interact with gliadin-specific CD4+ Th1 cells, which produce additional inflammatory cytokines (i.e. IFN-$\gamma$) [11, 15].

Genetic predisposition plays a strong role in development of celiac disease. There is known, frequent occurrence between familial generations. Birth cohort and population studies have shown that the most important genetic factors that drives risk for celiac disease are the class 2 human leukocyte antigen (HLA) genes, with an 80% concordance rate in homozygous twins [16–18]. Celiac disease is strongly associated with certain common HLA types. The two most important and common underlying genes thought to predispose to celiac disease consist of the following HLA class II genes: HLA-DQ2 (DQA1*05-DQB1*02) and HLA-DQ8 (DQA1*03-DQB1*0302) [19]. Overall, it is estimated that HLA-associated molecules contribute at least 40% of the heritable risk of celiac disease. There is a gene dosage to risk, and those with DQA1*05-DQB1*02 are five times more likely to have celiac than individuals with just a single allele of DQ2. More commonly, patients with celiac disease carry gene DQ2 (90%), and only about 5% to 7% carry DQ8. Indeed, most patients with celiac have the presence of either of these HLA types, and if neither is present, there is a negative predictive value of nearly 100% in excluding the diagnosis [20, 21]. Interestingly, many patients, even with high HLA-determined genetic risk, never develop celiac disease, suggesting the role of environmental and alternative immunological risk factors in disease development.

There are other less strongly associated non-HLA locus genes that may increase risk for celiac disease, though these are thought to contribute only about 14% to the genetic risk for the disease [20, 22]. Only very large studies, with thousands of patients, have found significant relative risk of these other non-HLA genes in developing celiac disease. The vast majority of the variants detected in non-HLA regions are in non-coding regions, and their exact influence on protein expression is not yet clear. Some genes however have been found to encode proteins including SH2B3 (a protective factor against bacterial infection) and RNAs including lnc13 RNA (expression control of other genes involved in the adaptive and innate immune systems) [23–25]. Other autoimmune diseases, such as type 1 diabetes, also share common genetic risk regions, including HLA-DQ [22]. Many have attempted to generate a risk score that combines the HLA and non-HLA regions, however, no such stratification means have been developed.

Recently, there is emerging data that a number of additional environmental factors are likely involved in the immune-response balance of celiac. These include the amount and quality of ingested gluten, the type and duration of wheat dough fermentation, early feeding of infants, the spectrum of intestinal microorganisms and how they change over time, intestinal infections, place of living and childhood growth, socioeconomic and smoking status, and stressors in general [26]. Ongoing studies are needed to determine the environmental factors and their specific influence on the balance between the immune response and tolerance to gluten. Studies are underway to determine if it is possible to reduce gluten antigenicity or eliminate toxic peptides from gluten as a method of primary prevention of celiac disease [27].

## Clinical Presentation

Celiac disease is recognized across all age ranges and presents with a spectrum of symptoms and associated conditions [28]. While it is thought that many patients may be asymptomatic, those who are symptomatic present with a wide variety of gastrointestinal and extra-intestinal symptoms. Indeed, the clinical manifestations of celiac disease vary and involve multiple organ symptoms.

Celiac disease is recognized as symptomatic disease (as above) and subclinical disease, which refers to patients who do not have symptoms and signs to trigger clinical suspicion of disease [29]. Symptomatic disease can be further divided into classical and non-classical disease. Any case with malabsorption is defined as classical disease and all other cases are non-classical. Overall, the presentation of diagnosed celiac disease has been changing. Diagnosis has seen a shift toward older individuals with milder disease, as opposed to children with severe disease as seen in the past [28]. This change has been attributed to increased awareness, better diagnostics, and earlier detection through serologic testing, and possibly later onset due to environmental factors such as increased wheat consumption [5, 7, 28–30].

In the past, celiac disease was described as a childhood disease consisting of malabsorption, weight loss, and diarrhea. Currently, these gastrointestinal symptoms are present in 30% to 50% of identified cases, the most common being diarrhea and flatulence. Diarrhea is the hallmark symptom of celiac disease. More recently, the proportion of patients with celiac disease who present with diarrhea has decreased, owing to earlier diagnosis by serologic testing [7]. Other symptoms typically include steatorrhea, dyspepsia, bloating, and abdominal pain [31]. Many patients are vulnerable to fat malabsorption, which results in steatorrhea [32]. Abdominal pain and bloating may be anywhere from mild to severe, observed in 40% to 50% of patients [8]. Hepatobiliary complications include elevated transaminases levels in 20% to 40% of adults at time of initial diagnosis, resolved with gluten-free diet. Rarer hepatobiliary manifestations include primary biliary cirrhosis, autoimmune hepatitis, or primary sclerosing cholangitis [33, 34]. Despite the well characterized gastrointestinal symptoms that can occur in celiac disease, individual symptoms lack specificity [35].

Many extra-intestinal symptoms are directly or indirectly caused by malabsorption of calories; however, the autoimmune process appears to be responsible for at least some of the extra-intestinal manifestations. Weight loss occurs in 40% to 50% of patients due to inadequate absorption of calories from food, and chronic fatigue is a common associated manifestation [8]. Weight loss, malabsorption, and other multifactorial causes lead to extra-intestinal clinical manifestations in children adults that are unique.

Children may present with failure to thrive with inadequate gains in weight and height [36]. Short stature is the most common extra-intestinal presentation of celiac disease in children, sometimes being the only clinical sign. Malabsorption in addition to dysfunction of growth hormone, insulin-like growth factor, and pro-inflammatory cytokines (IL-6, TNF-a) are thought to play roles [37]. Delayed puberty is a common finding due to hypogonadism in girls and androgen resistance in boys [38]. Anemia is only present in 15% of the celiac pediatric population, most frequently due to iron (ineffective iron absorption in the duodenal mucosa), vitamin B12, and folate deficiencies [39]. Majority of children can have complete recovery of their anemia by strictly adhering to the gluten-free diet [40]. The bone manifestations include osteopenia (75%) and osteoporosis (10–30%) [41]. This is due to the duodenal mucosa being the site where most Vitamin D and calcium are absorbed, subsequently causing increase in parathyroid hormone with bone turnover [42]. These bone sequelae are often reversed with gluten-free adherence in addition to calcium-fortified foods, and vitamin D metabolites [43]. A number of neurologic manifestations are associated with celiac in children, the most common being headache (20%) [44]. Rarely, they may experience ataxia and neuropathy. Seizures have also been reported. These deficits have been seen to occur mostly due to vitamin deficiencies (E, B12, D) or micronutrients (magnesium) [45]. Enamel defects can be seen, and when the defect affects permanent teeth, there is no improvement upon the induction of a gluten-free diet [46].

Adults have a different profile of extra-intestinal manifestations. Presentation with anemia is more common in adults than in children. Most commonly anemia is found to be secondary to iron deficiency (malabsorption and/or occult bleeding), anemia of chronic disease, and vitamin/micronutrient deficiencies (B12, folate, fat-soluble vitamins) [47, 48]. These adults require nutritional supplementation. Hyposplenism may be seen in those with concomitant autoimmune disorders. Adults may also have other hematologic findings including IgA deficiency, low cholesterol, platelet disorders, venous thromboembolism, and lymphoma (particularly intestinal) [49]. Severe disease may result in abnormal bleeding or bruising (vitamin K deficiency). Patients may experience symptoms of vitamin D deficiency, including muscle cramps and pain/tenderness in bones. Adults may have a history of fractures resulting from osteoporosis [36]. Dermatitis herpetiformis is an autoimmune response to ingested gluten that manifests as a papulovesicular rash on extensor surfaces, and skin biopsy reveals granular immunoglobulin A deposits at the dermal-epidermal junction of the affected skin [50–53]. Oral findings include aphthous ulcers, cheilosis, lichen planus, and atrophic glossitis [54, 55]. As in children, gait ataxia, neuropathy, and headaches may be seen. Some women may experience decreased fertility as a long-term side effect. Some may experience recurrent miscarriages, and infants born to women with celiac are at risk for exhibiting low birth weight, increased perinatal mortality rate, and may breastfeed for shorter intervals

[6, 11]. Delayed menarche, secondary amenorrhea, and earlier menopause are reported.

Concurrent autoimmune conditions can be found in 35% of celiac patients. Often individuals with celiac disease are more likely to have more than one autoimmune disease [56]. Hashimoto's thyroiditis is the most commonly associated autoimmune disorder, of whom 2.7% have celiac disease [57]. Psoriasis is the second most commonly associated autoimmune condition (4.3%), followed by T1DM, which is found in 4% of cases of celiac, followed by Sjogren's syndrome (2.4%) [28, 47, 56, 58].

## Physical Examination Findings

Physical examination findings may be important in supporting the diagnosis of celiac disease. Some patients have unremarkable examination findings, whereas those with severe disease may have extraordinary findings, as well as evidence of systemic malabsorption. Tympanic abdomen occurs in 40% to 50% of patients [8]. Signs of malabsorption and protein-calorie malnutrition may present with weight loss, muscle wasting, and edema due to hypoproteinemia. Signs of vitamin deficiencies (due to malabsorption) may present as pallor associated with iron deficiency or folate deficiency anemia; there may also be evidence of fractures or reduced bone density due to osteoporosis [7]. Less common signs include rashes, i.e. aphthous ulcers. Dermatitis herpetiformis may be seen as an eruption of blisters on the scalp, buttocks, and/or extensor surfaces of knees and elbows, and when found is diagnostic of celiac disease [8]. Although not always associated with intestinal manifestations, many patients display vitamin malabsorption and intestinal villous atrophy [59]. Physical examination may also reveal ataxia and/or neuropathy, typically sensory symptoms greater than motor [32].

Children may have similar but age-unique clinical presentations. They may similarly have abdominal distension, weight loss, and muscle wasting due to malabsorption [60]. In older children, the sequelae of malabsorption may present with delayed puberty and short stature. Neurologic symptoms may be seen, which are largely consequential in this vulnerable age group. In fact, the pediatric population is 2.5 times more susceptible to neurologic disorders than older populations. These include hypotonia, developmental delay, learning and attention deficits, and cerebellar symptoms (impaired coordination and unsteady gait) [61]. As mentioned previously, there may be evidence of rickets, with bone fractures, dental deformities such as enamel defects, and skeletal deformities (i.e. genu varum, rachitic rosary, misshapen skull).

# Diagnosis of Celiac Disease

Those who display the classical symptoms and physical examination findings for celiac disease should be tested, based on clinical suspicion of the evaluating physician. There is a lack of evidence for mass screening, and the US Preventive Services Task Force recently released a statement against testing for celiac disease in asymptomatic individuals, owing to the lack of strong benefit [28]. Of note, patients with villous atrophy and negative celiac disease serologies pose diagnostic and therapeutic dilemma; the optimal methods for screening and management are unknown but recommend surveillance endoscopies and consideration of alternative diagnoses as patients with villous atrophy are at risk for complications [62]. More methods are needed to identify who should be tested for celiac disease, and case finding remains the recommended strategy.

Initial assessment of celiac disease consists of history and physical examination. Further evaluation involves serologic testing, and follow-up with intestinal biopsy based on serologic testing results. In approximately 10% of cases, diagnosis is obscured by lack of concordance among serologic, clinical, and histologic findings. Most importantly, diagnostic testing must occur while the patient's diet contains gluten. It is recommended that patients ingest at minimum three grams of gluten per day for two weeks prior to undergoing diagnostic studies [63]. Antibodies disappear in patients practicing a gluten-free diet, therefore if a patient has not been on a gluten diet, baseline serologic testing should be obtained. If this is negative, HLA typing can be performed to check for genetic markers [64]. Positive genetic testing should potentiate a gluten challenge [64].

Serologic testing is used as the screening tool for celiac, since endoscopy and biopsy are significantly more invasive and expensive. Testing for sensitive and specific antibody targets against endomysium, TTG, and synthetic deamidated gliadin peptides is commonly used. While the international guidelines for testing differ, TTG-IgA is the highest recommended screening test, given its great sensitivity. Of note, more recent literature shows that sensitivity may not be as high as previously estimated; therefore, sequential testing wit hTTg-IgA, EMA, or DGP-IgG may be more sensitive screening tests [64–66].

In the adult population, endoscopy with small intestinal biopsy is the gold standard and required for final diagnosis [67]. On endoscopy, majority of celiac disease cases reveal patchy mucosal changes, with more significant injury in the proximal intestine [68]. About 10% of patients will have changes in the duodenal bulb only. The characteristic histologic changes consistent with celiac disease involve the superficial intestinal mucosa, with increased intraepithelial lymphocytes, crypt elongation (hyperplasia or hypertrophy), and loss of villus height in the form of partial or complete villous atrophy [10]. The lamina propria experiences an infiltrate of plasma and lymphocytic cells (predominantly CD8+ T cells), which localize in the tips of villi [69]. Further, the degree of change in the villus architecture as compared to crypt elongation is called the villous-height-to-crypt-depth. Decreasing values in villous-height-to-crypt-depth ratio indicate greater histologic changes [10, 70].

There are instances in which serologic and endoscopic or biopsy results do not coincide. Clinicians may be faced with patients who have villus atrophy on duodenal biopsy but negative serology [71]. These cases can represent either an alternative diagnosis or seronegative celiac disease. The TTG antibodies have been found in the small bowel mucosa of seronegative cases, leading to the hypothesis that these antibodies are unable to pass into circulation [72]. There are instances in which serologies may be negative while histology and clinical presentation are consistent with celiac disease. Diagnosis of seronegative celiac disease in this manner requires exclusion of alternative causes of villous atrophy, response to a gluten-free diet, and permissive HLA typing. Negative serologies in patients with celiac disease may be due to any one of the following: 1) patients with IgA deficiency (tTG-IgA serology will be falsely negative) 2) those already on a gluten free diet 3) false negative test results (while the antibodies have very high sensitivity, this is still possible). Alternative diagnosis on the differential of celiac disease include irritable bowel syndrome, small intestinal bacterial overgrowth, lactose intolerance, chronic pancreatitis, microscopic colitis, and inflammatory bowel disease. Clinical context and additional diagnostic data must be taken into consideration when invoking such alternative diagnoses. Furthermore, those who are diagnosed with true seronegative celiac may experience more severe disease, such as refractory celiac disease, defined as is resistant or unresponsive to at least 12 months of treatment with a strict gluten-free diet. The converse situation is also possible, with positive serology and normal biopsy or increased intraepithelial lymphocytes with no atrophy [69]. These situations may reflect celiac disease with poor tissue sampling, latent celiac disease or false-positive serologic test result. HLA typing may rule out celiac disease if negative. A trial of gluten-free diet can also be considered to further characterize whether or not there is resolution of symptoms in those with difficulty in making the diagnosis. However, an empiric trial of a gluten-free diet without a biopsy is not recommended because symptoms of other disorders (e.g., irritable bowel syndrome, reflux, functional dyspepsia) can improve in patients following this diet. One study noted that the positive predictive value of a beneficial response from eliminating gluten in the diet was only 36% [73].

# Video Capsule Endoscopy and Enteroscopy in Celiac Disease

Video capsule endoscopy (VCE) is a minimally invasive form of examination that produces highly magnified views of the entire small bowel mucosa. The role of VCE in celiac disease is still evolving [74–76]. The advantage over standard endoscopy involves a highly magnified view of the mucosa for better detection of villous changes, while the disadvantage is the lack of intestinal sampling. While duodenal biopsy is the gold standard for diagnosis of celiac disease, some patients have patchy villous atrophy, that may be poorly detected on traditional endoscopy. In this way, VCE's ability to examine the entire small bowel mucosa increases sensitivity for diagnosis [11]. Some studies have shown that a potential new application for VCE is noninvasive evaluation of the response to a gluten-free diet [75, 76]. Currently, the European Society of Gastrointestinal Endoscopy guidelines state that there is currently no role for the use of VCE to evaluate the extent of disease or monitor the response to a gluten free diet, although these guidelines might change with emerging research in the field [77].

Celiac disease involves predominantly the proximal portion of the small bowel, given that it is the first site of gluten exposure. Inflammation is most commonly found in the duodenum, which is easily reached by standard endoscopy for diagnosis. Rarely, celiac disease spares the duodenum and involves the jejunum alone [78]. In such patients, with negative duodenal biopsy but high clinical suspicion of disease, enteroscopy is required for diagnosis. Enteroscopy may also be very useful in evaluating the complications of disease. For example, celiac disease is associated with an increased risk for gastrointestinal cancers that include adenocarcinoma of the small bowel, often more easily detected with enteroscopy than endoscopy [79]. Enteroscopy is also used for diagnosis and management of refractory celiac disease [80, 81].

# Follow-Up of Celiac Disease

The only effective treatment for celiac disease is complete removal of gluten from the diet, and it is key that patients follow a strict gluten-free diet (GFD), which results in symptomatic, serologic, and histologic remission in most patients [82]. The management and follow-up of patients with celiac disease requires multidisciplinary care [82].

Follow-up is tightly related to adherence of GFD. It is known that GFD leads to significant improvement in symptoms, normalization of serologic measures, and increase in quality of life for many patients. However, it is known that patients may find it difficult to adhere to the GFD, and there are many concerns surrounding this topic that require close attention from the team of providers [83]. On a broad scale, children follow up with a pediatric gastroenterologist even after diagnosis; whereas adults may often follow-up with their primary care providers after initial diagnosis by gastroenterologist and instead return to gastroenterology at yearly interventions or at time of complication [84, 85]. Dieticians play an integral role in maintaining patient adherence, by providing them the knowledge about modifying and personalizing the GFD. They help assessing nutritional status, identifying macro- and micronutrient deficiencies/excesses, analyze eating habits, provide information, advise, and education, and reinforce dietary counseling [82].

Nutritional deficiencies usually present during time of celiac diagnosis are important to follow up closely, particularly in children and adolescents. Nutritional deficiencies that require close follow-up include those in iron, calcium, vitamin B12, folate [86]. Furthermore, pediatric gastroenterologists should closely follow height and weight as an essential marker of success of the GFD in children and adolescents. Further, patient-reported symptoms and quality of life should be carefully assessed in this population as well [87]. Children who are lost to follow-up are more frequently nonadherent to GFD and will have more severe disease with subsequent complications [88]. The use of serology to monitor this population is limited but still should be part of the overall follow up of a patient with celiac disease. The use of systematic endoscopy and biopsy is avoided given the invasive nature and requirement for general anesthesia [89, 90].

Adults require holistic follow-up, given that the GFD pervades not only their medical lives, but also their social and professional activities. Adults on GFD may be asymptomatic, but some may have relapse or be persistently symptomatic [91]. Follow-up of adult patients requires thorough evaluation of symptoms, performance of general laboratory tests (i.e. complete blood count, serum iron, vitamin B12, folic acid, calcium, vitamin d), and celiac disease serology. DXA scanning should be performed at baseline and compared at intervals; abnormalities may require mineral supplementation and in some cases referral to a specialist. Further, vaccination against *pneumococci*, *haemophilusinfluenza*, and *meningococci* are strongly recommended [84].

Some gastroenterologists use mucosal healing as a marker of follow-up in those adherent to the GFD, largely to assess intestinal recovery and exclusion of malignancies [33]. Studies have shown varying results and conclusions with regard to the need for follow-up biopsies [65, 92, 93]. For some patients, intestinal biopsies and mucosal evaluation may not accurately reflect clinical status as healing and histological recovery may be delayed relative to symptomatic improvement, even in those who are strictly adherent [4]. Alternatively, there is some evidence that continued mucosal damage on endoscopy and biopsy may be associated with clinical deterioration, increased mortality, and complications such as bone fractures and onset of lymphoma [39, 40, 94]. Follow-up intestinal biopsies in those who are persistently symptomatic may also be used to exclude refractory celiac disease. In combining the evidence so far, it seems that the decision to follow-up biopsy should be based mostly on expert decisions, and likely in those who are persistently symptomatic with adherence to the GFD, given possibility for poor outcomes [92, 93].

There are new tools that have emerged for patients who may be unaware of dietary indiscretion and have continuing symptoms. These include the new quantitative ELISA (for stool) and quantitative immune-chromotography (for urine), which assess gluten immunogenic peptides [95, 96]. These point-of-care tests are simple and can be used at home or in a physician's office. However, the utility of such measures are currently unclear and there is not enough evidence for frequent, accurate use.

# Conclusion

Celiac disease is the most common immune-mediated enteropathy. Environmental and dietary factors amongst genetic predisposition plays a significant role in the disease process of celiac disease. Celiac disease is recognized along a wide spectrum of ages, and patients may experiences classical intestinal as well as extra-intestinal disease manifestations. Among those with consistent clinical symptoms and physical examination, serologic testing may be used as a screening tool, however endoscopy with small intestinal biopsy is the gold standard and required for final diagnosis [67]. The only effective treatment for celiac disease is complete removal of gluten from the diet, which results in symptomatic, serologic, and histologic remission in most patients. The management and follow-up celiac disease requires multidisciplinary care. Ongoing studies aim to advance understanding in the pathogenesis of celiac disease that could enable preventive strategies for patients at high risk of disease development. Current and future investigations are aspiring to develop non-dietary therapies, particularly for individuals who find adhering to the gluten-free diet challenging [97].

# References

1. Lebwohl B, Sanders DS, Green PHR. Coeliac disease. Lancet. 2018;391(10115):70–81.
2. HAAS SV. Celiac disease, its specific treatment and cure without nutritional relapse. JAMA. 1932;99:448–52.
3. Booth C. History of coeliac disease. BMJ. 1989;297(6664):1646–9.
4. Dicke WK, Weijers HA, Van De Kamer JH. Coeliac disease. II. The presence in wheat of a factor having a deleterious effect in cases of coeliac disease. Acta Paediatr. 1953;42(1):34–42.
5. Van De Kamer JH, Weijers HA, Dicke WK. Coeliac disease. IV. An investigation into the injurious constituents of wheat in connection with their action on patients with coeliac disease. Acta Paediatr. 1953;42(3):223–31.
6. Singh P, Arora A, Strand TA, Leffler DA, Catassi C, Green PH, et al. Global prevalence of celiac disease: systematic review and meta-analysis. Clin Gastroenterol Hepatol. 2018;16(6):823–36. e2
7. Lo W, Sano K, Lebwohl B, Diamond B, Green PH. Changing presentation of adult celiac disease. Dig Dis Sci. 2003;48(2):395–8.
8. Fasano A, Catassi C. Clinical practice. Celiac disease. N Engl J Med. 2012;367(25):2419–26.
9. Sapone A, Bai JC, Ciacci C, Dolinsek J, Green PH, Hadjivassiliou M, et al. Spectrum of gluten-related disorders: consensus on new nomenclature and classification. BMC Med. 2012;10:13.
10. Husby S, Olsson C, Ivarsson A. Celiac disease and risk management of gluten. In: Risk management for food allergy. Cambridge, MA: Academic Press; 2014. p. 129–52.
11. Green PH, Cellier C. Celiac disease. N Engl J Med. 2007;357(17):1731–43.
12. Dieterich W, Ehnis T, Bauer M, Donner P, Volta U, Riecken EO, et al. Identification of tissue transglutaminase as the autoantigen of celiac disease. Nat Med. 1997;3(7):797–801.
13. Maiuri L, Ciacci C, Ricciardelli I, Vacca L, Raia V, Auricchio S, et al. Association between innate response to gliadin and activation of pathogenic T cells in coeliac disease. Lancet. 2003;362(9377):30–7.

14. Mention JJ, Ben Ahmed M, Begue B, Barbe U, Verkarre V, Asnafi V, et al. Interleukin 15: a key to disrupted intraepithelial lymphocyte homeostasis and lymphomagenesis in celiac disease. Gastroenterology. 2003;125(3):730–45.

15. Schuppan D, Junker Y, Barisani D. Celiac disease: from pathogenesis to novel therapies. Gastroenterology. 2009;137(6):1912–33.

16. Greco L, Romino R, Coto I, Di Cosmo N, Percopo S, Maglio M, et al. The first large population based twin study of coeliac disease. Gut. 2002;50(5):624–8.

17. Kuja-Halkola R, Lebwohl B, Halfvarson J, Wijmenga C, Magnusson PK, Ludvigsson JF. Heritability of non-HLA genetics in coeliac disease: a population-based study in 107 000 twins. Gut. 2016;65(11):1793–8.

18. Nistico L, Fagnani C, Coto I, Percopo S, Cotichini R, Limongelli MG, et al. Concordance, disease progression, and heritability of coeliac disease in Italian twins. Gut. 2006;55(6):803–8.

19. Sollid LM, Lie BA. Celiac disease genetics: current concepts and practical applications. Clin Gastroenterol Hepatol. 2005;3(9):843–51.

20. Romanos J, van Diemen CC, Nolte IM, Trynka G, Zhernakova A, Fu J, et al. Analysis of HLA and non-HLA alleles can identify individuals at high risk for celiac disease. Gastroenterology. 2009;137(3):834–40. 40 e1–3

21. Kaukinen K, Partanen J, Maki M, Collin P. HLA-DQ typing in the diagnosis of celiac disease. Am J Gastroenterol. 2002;97(3):695–9.

22. Hunt KA, Zhernakova A, Turner G, Heap GA, Franke L, Bruinenberg M, et al. Newly identified genetic risk variants for celiac disease related to the immune response. Nat Genet. 2008;40(4):395–402.

23. Zhernakova A, Elbers CC, Ferwerda B, Romanos J, Trynka G, Dubois PC, et al. Evolutionary and functional analysis of celiac risk loci reveals SH2B3 as a protective factor against bacterial infection. Am J Hum Genet. 2010;86(6):970–7.

24. Castellanos-Rubio A, Fernandez-Jimenez N, Kratchmarov R, Luo X, Bhagat G, Green PH, et al. A long noncoding RNA associated with susceptibility to celiac disease. Science. 2016;352(6281):91–5.

25. Castellanos-Rubio A, Santin I, Irastorza I, Castano L, Carlos Vitoria J, Ramon Bilbao J. TH17 (and TH1) signatures of intestinal biopsies of CD patients in response to gliadin. Autoimmunity. 2009;42(1):69–73.

26. Lionetti E, Catassi C. New clues in celiac disease epidemiology, pathogenesis, clinical manifestations, and treatment. Int Rev Immunol. 2011;30(4):219–31.

27. Panel NI-SE, Boyce JA, Assa'ad A, Burks AW, Jones SM, Sampson HA, et al. Guidelines for the diagnosis and management of food allergy in the United States: report of the NIAID-sponsored expert panel. J Allergy Clin Immunol. 2010;126(6 Suppl):S1–58.

28. Dominguez Castro P, Harkin G, Hussey M, Christopher B, Kiat C, Liong Chin J, et al. Changes in presentation of celiac disease in Ireland from the 1960s to 2015. Clin Gastroenterol Hepatol. 2017;15(6):864–71. e3

29. Ludvigsson JF, Leffler DA, Bai JC, Biagi F, Fasano A, Green PH, et al. The Oslo definitions for coeliac disease and related terms. Gut. 2013;62(1):43–52.

30. Ramakrishna BS, Makharia GK, Chetri K, Dutta S, Mathur P, Ahuja V, et al. Prevalence of adult celiac disease in India: regional variations and associations. Am J Gastroenterol. 2016;111(1):115–23.

31. Maglione MA, Okunogbe A, Ewing B, Grant S, Newberry SJ, Motala A, et al. Diagnosis of celiac disease. Rockville, MD: AHRQ Comparative Effectiveness Reviews; 2016.

32. Green PH. The many faces of celiac disease: clinical presentation of celiac disease in the adult population. Gastroenterology. 2005;128(4 Suppl 1):S74–8.

33. Rubio-Tapia A, Murray JA. The liver in celiac disease. Hepatology. 2007;46(5):1650–8.

34. Sainsbury A, Sanders DS, Ford AC. Meta-analysis: coeliac disease and hypertransaminasaemia. Aliment Pharmacol Ther. 2011;34(1):33–40.

35. Vogelsang H, Genser D, Wyatt J, Lochs H, Ferenci P, Granditsch G, et al. Screening for celiac disease: a prospective study on the value of noninvasive tests. Am J Gastroenterol. 1995;90(3):394–8.

36. Khatib M, Baker RD, Ly EK, Kozielski R, Baker SS. Presenting pattern of pediatric celiac disease. J Pediatr Gastroenterol Nutr. 2016;62(1):60–3.

37. Meazza C, Pagani S, Laarej K, Cantoni F, Civallero P, Boncimino A, et al. Short stature in children with coeliac disease. Pediatr Endocrinol Rev. 2009;6(4):457–63.

38. Street ME, Volta C, Ziveri MA, Zanacca C, Banchini G, Viani I, et al. Changes and relationships of IGFS and IGFBPS and cytokines in coeliac disease at diagnosis and on gluten-free diet. Clin Endocrinol. 2008;68(1):22–8.

39. Nurminen S, Kivela L, Huhtala H, Kaukinen K, Kurppa K. Extraintestinal manifestations were common in children with coeliac disease and were more prevalent in patients with more severe clinical and histological presentation. Acta Paediatr. 2019;108(4):681–7.

40. Jericho H, Sansotta N, Guandalini S. Extraintestinal manifestations of celiac disease: effectiveness of the gluten-free diet. J Pediatr Gastroenterol Nutr. 2017;65(1):75–9.

41. Pantaleoni S, Luchino M, Adriani A, Pellicano R, Stradella D, Ribaldone DG, et al. Bone mineral density at diagnosis of celiac disease and after 1 year of gluten-free diet. ScientificWorldJournal. 2014;2014:173082.

42. Keaveny AP, Freaney R, McKenna MJ, Masterson J, O'Donoghue DP. Bone remodeling indices and secondary hyperparathyroidism in celiac disease. Am J Gastroenterol. 1996;91(6):1226–31.

43. Krupa-Kozak U, Markiewicz LH, Lamparski G, Juskiewicz J. Administration of inulin-supplemented gluten-free diet modified calcium absorption and caecal microbiota in rats in a calcium-dependent manner. Nutrients. 2017;9(7):702.

44. Casella G, Bordo BM, Schalling R, Villanacci V, Salemme M, Di Bella C, et al. Neurological disorders and celiac disease. Minerva Gastroenterol Dietol. 2016;62(2):197–206.

45. Ludvigsson JF, Zingone F, Tomson T, Ekbom A, Ciacci C. Increased risk of epilepsy in biopsy-verified celiac disease: a population-based cohort study. Neurology. 2012;78(18):1401–7.

46. Farmakis E, Puntis JW, Toumba KJ. Enamel defects in children with coeliac disease. Eur J Paediatr Dent. 2005;6(3):129–32.

47. Volta U, Caio G, Stanghellini V, De Giorgio R. The changing clinical profile of celiac disease: a 15-year experience (1998-2012) in an Italian referral center. BMC Gastroenterol. 2014;14:194.

48. Schosler L, Christensen LA, Hvas CL. Symptoms and findings in adult-onset celiac disease in a historical Danish patient cohort. Scand J Gastroenterol. 2016;51(3):288–94.

49. Halfdanarson TR, Litzow MR, Murray JA. Hematologic manifestations of celiac disease. Blood. 2007;109(2):412–21.

50. Bolotin D, Petronic-Rosic V. Dermatitis herpetiformis. Part I. Epidemiology, pathogenesis, and clinical presentation. J Am Acad Dermatol. 2011;64(6):1017–24. quiz 25–6

51. Collin P, Reunala T. Recognition and management of the cutaneous manifestations of celiac disease: a guide for dermatologists. Am J Clin Dermatol. 2003;4(1):13–20.

52. Gawkrodger DJ, Blackwell JN, Gilmour HM, Rifkind EA, Heading RC, Barnetson RS. Dermatitis herpetiformis: diagnosis, diet and demography. Gut. 1984;25(2):151–7.

53. Gregory B, Ho VC. Cutaneous manifestations of gastrointestinal disorders. Part II. J Am Acad Dermatol. 1992;26(3 Pt 2):371–83.

54. Pastore L, Carroccio A, Compilato D, Panzarella V, Serpico R, Lo Muzio L. Oral manifestations of celiac disease. J Clin Gastroenterol. 2008;42(3):224–32.

55. Rashid M, Zarkadas M, Anca A, Limeback H. Oral manifestations of celiac disease: a clinical guide for dentists. J Can Dent Assoc. 2011;77:b39.

56. Bibbo S, Pes GM, Usai-Satta P, Salis R, Soro S, Quarta Colosso BM, et al. Chronic autoimmune disorders are increased in coeliac disease: a case-control study. Medicine (Baltimore). 2017;96(47):e8562.

57. Roy A, Laszkowska M, Sundstrom J, Lebwohl B, Green PH, Kampe O, et al. Prevalence of celiac disease in patients with autoimmune thyroid disease: a meta-analysis. Thyroid. 2016;26(7):880–90.
58. Elfsrom P, Sundström J, Ludvigsson JF. Systematic review with meta-analysis: associations between coeliac disease and type 1 diabetes. Ailment Pharmacol Ther. 2014;40(10):1123–32.
59. Krishnareddy S, Lewis SK, Green PH. Dermatitis herpetiformis: clinical presentations are independent of manifestations of celiac disease. Am J Clin Dermatol. 2014;15(1):51–6.
60. Green PH, Jabri B. Coeliac disease. Lancet. 2003;362(9381):383–91.
61. Zelnik N, Pacht A, Obeid R, Lerner A. Range of neurologic disorders in patients with celiac disease. Pediatrics. 2004;113(6):1672–6.
62. Leonard MM, Lebwohl B, Rubio-Tapia A, Biagi F. AGA clinical practice update on the evaluation and management of seronegative enteropathies: expert review. Gastroenterology. 2021;160:437–44.
63. Leffler D, Schuppan D, Pallav K, Najarian R, Goldsmith JD, Hansen J, et al. Kinetics of the histological, serological and symptomatic responses to gluten challenge in adults with coeliac disease. Gut. 2013;62(7):996–1004.
64. Lau MS, Sanders DS. Optimizing the diagnosis of celiac disease. Curr Opin Gastroenterol. 2017;33(3):173–80.
65. Ludvigsson JF, Bai JC, Biagi F, Card TR, Ciacci C, Ciclitira PJ, et al. Diagnosis and management of adult coeliac disease: guidelines from the British Society of Gastroenterology. Gut. 2014;63(8):1210–28.
66. Kumar VJ-C, M.; Sulej, J.; Karnewska, K.; Farrell, T.; Jablonska, S. Celiac disease and immunoglobulin A deficiency: how effective are the serological methods of diagnosis? Clin Diagn Lab Immunol. 2002;9(6):1295–300.
67. Latorre M, Lagana SM, Freedberg DE, Lewis SK, Lebwohl B, Bhagat G, et al. Endoscopic biopsy technique in the diagnosis of celiac disease: one bite or two? Gastrointest Endosc. 2015;81(5):1228–33.
68. Oberhuber G. Histopathology of celiac disease. Biomed Pharmacother. 2000;54(7):368–72.
69. Salmi TT, Collin P, Korponay-Szabo IR, Laurila K, Partanen J, Huhtala H, et al. Endomysial antibody-negative celiac disease: clinical characteristics and intestinal autoantibody deposits. Gut. 2006;55(12):1746–53.
70. Barada K, Habib RH, Malli A, Hashash JG, Halawi H, Maasri K, et al. Prediction of celiac disease at endoscopy. Endoscopy. 2014;46(2):110–9.
71. Lewis NR, Scott BB. Systematic review: the use of serology to exclude or diagnose coeliac disease (a comparison of the endomysial and tissue transglutaminase antibody tests). Aliment Pharmacol Ther. 2006;24(1):47–54.
72. Amarri S, Alvisi P, De Giorgio R, Gelli MC, Cicola R, Tovoli F, et al. Antibodies to deamidated gliadin peptides: an accurate predictor of coeliac disease in infancy. J Clin Immunol. 2013;33(5):1027–30.
73. Campanella J, Biagi F, Bianchi PI, Zanellati G, Marchese A, Corazza GR. Clinical response to gluten withdrawal is not an indicator of coeliac disease. Scand J Gastroenterol. 2008;43(11):1311–4.
74. Lewis SK, Semrad CE. Capsule endoscopy and Enteroscopy in celiac disease. Gastroenterol Clin N Am. 2019;48(1):73–84.
75. Chang MS, Rubin M, Lewis SK, Green PH. Diagnosing celiac disease by video capsule endoscopy (VCE) when esophagogastroduodenoscopy (EGD) and biopsy is unable to provide a diagnosis: a case series. BMC Gastroenterol. 2012;12:90.
76. Rondonotti E, Paggi S. Videocapsule endoscopy in celiac disease: indications and timing. Dig Dis. 2015;33(2):244–51.
77. Pennazio M, Spada C, Eliakim R, Keuchel M, May A, Mulder CJ, et al. Small-bowel capsule endoscopy and device-assisted enteroscopy for diagnosis and treatment of small-bowel disorders: European Society of Gastrointestinal Endoscopy (ESGE) clinical guideline. Endoscopy. 2015;47(4):352–76.

78. Valitutti F, Di Nardo G, Barbato M, Aloi M, Celletti I, Trovato CM, et al. Mapping histologic patchiness of celiac disease by push enteroscopy. Gastrointest Endosc. 2014;79(1):95–100.
79. Hadithi M, Al-toma A, Oudejans J, van Bodegraven AA, Mulder CJ, Jacobs M. The value of double-balloon Enteroscopy in patients with refractory celiac disease. Am J Gastroenterol. 2007;102:987–96.
80. Tomba C, Elli L, Bardella MT, Soncini M, Contiero P, Roncoroni L, et al. Enteroscopy for the early detection of small bowel tumours in at-risk celiac patients. Dig Liver Dis. 2014;46(5):400–4.
81. Elli L, Casazza G, Locatelli M, Branchi F, Ferretti F, Conte D, et al. Use of enteroscopy for the detection of malignant and premalignant lesions of the small bowel in complicated celiac disease: a meta-analysis. Gastrointest Endosc. 2017;86(2):264–73. e1
82. See JA, Kaukinen K, Makharia GK, Gibson PR, Murray JA. Practical insights into gluten-free diets. Nat Rev Gastroenterol Hepatol. 2015;12(10):580–91.
83. Mahadev S, Murray JA, Wu TT, Chandan VS, Torbenson MS, Kelly CP, et al. Factors associated with villus atrophy in symptomatic coeliac disease patients on a gluten-free diet. Aliment Pharmacol Ther. 2017;45(8):1084–93.
84. Hall NJ, Rubin G, Charnock A. Systematic review: adherence to a gluten-free diet in adult patients with coeliac disease. Aliment Pharmacol Ther. 2009;30(4):315–30.
85. Cohen ME, Jaffe A, Strauch CB, Lewis SK, Lebwohl B, Green PHR. Determinants of follow-up care for patients with celiac disease. J Clin Gastroenterol. 2018;52(9):784–8.
86. Wessels MM, van V, II, Vriezinga SL, Putter H, Rings EH, Mearin ML. Complementary serologic investigations in children with celiac disease is unnecessary during follow-up. J Pediatr. 2016;169:55–60.
87. Ukkola A, Maki M, Kurppa K, Collin P, Huhtala H, Kekkonen L, et al. Patients' experiences and perceptions of living with coeliac disease - implications for optimizing care. J Gastrointestin Liver Dis. 2012;21(1):17–22.
88. De Palma G, Nadal I, Medina M, Donat E, Ribes-Koninckx C, Calabuig M, et al. Intestinal dysbiosis and reduced immunoglobulin-coated bacteria associated with coeliac disease in children. BMC Microbiol. 2010;10:63.
89. Guandalini S, Newland C. Can we really skip the biopsy in diagnosing symptomatic children with celiac disease. J Pediatr Gastroenterol Nutr. 2013;57(4):e24.
90. Vecsei E, Steinwendner S, Kogler H, Innerhofer A, Hammer K, Haas OA, et al. Follow-up of pediatric celiac disease: value of antibodies in predicting mucosal healing, a prospective cohort study. BMC Gastroenterol. 2014;14:28.
91. Bai JC, Fried M, Corazza GR, Schuppan D, Farthing M, Catassi C, et al. World gastroenterology organisation global guidelines on celiac disease. J Clin Gastroenterol. 2013;47(2):121–6.
92. Lebwohl B, Granath F, Ekbom A, Smedby KE, Murray JA, Neugut AI, et al. Mucosal healing and risk for lymphoproliferative malignancy in celiac disease: a population-based cohort study. Ann Intern Med. 2013;159(3):169–75.
93. Comino I, Real A, Vivas S, Siglez MA, Caminero A, Nistal E, et al. Monitoring of gluten-free diet compliance in celiac patients by assessment of gliadin 33-mer equivalent epitopes in feces. Am J Clin Nutr. 2012;95(3):670–7.
94. Lebwohl B, Murray JA, Rubio-Tapia A, Green PHR, Ludvigsson JF. Predictors of persistent villous atrophy in coeliac disease: a population-based study. Aliment Pharmacol Ther. 2014;39(5):488–95.
95. Moreno ML, Cebolla A, Munoz-Suano A, Carrillo-Carrion C, Comino I, Pizarro A, et al. Detection of gluten immunogenic peptides in the urine of patients with coeliac disease reveals transgressions in the gluten-free diet and incomplete mucosal healing. Gut. 2017;66(2):250–7.
96. Syage JA, Kelly CP, Dickason MA, Ramirez AC, Leon F, Dominguez R, et al. Determination of gluten consumption in celiac disease patients on a gluten-free diet. Am J Clin Nutr. 2018;107(2):201–7.
97. Kivela L, Caminero A, Leffler DA, Pinto-Sanchez MI, Tye-Din AJ, Lindfors K. Current and emerging therapies for coeliac disease. Nat Rev Gastroenterol Hepatol. 2021;18(3):181–95.

# Mechanisms of Lymphomagenesis in Celiac Disease: Lessons for Therapy

Sascha Cording, Sofia Berrabah, Ludovic Lhermitte, Georgia Malamut, and Nadine Cerf-Bensussan

## Introduction

Lymphomas are rare but characteristic and most severe complications of celiac disease (CeD). Their pathophysiology illustrates the driving role of inflammation in intestinal lymphomagenesis, while their mutational landscape reveals the importance of the JAK1-STAT3 pathway in the intestine as well as the overlap between the mechanisms that underlie autoimmunity and lymphocyte transformation. After summarizing the studies that have identified the association between CeD and lymphomas and their origin from intraepithelial lymphocytes, we review recent work that provides precise insight into the scenario through which chronic inflammation promotes lymphoma development with or without the intermediary step of intraepithelial lymphoma that defines type 2 refractory CeD (RCD2).

S. Cording · S. Berrabah
Université de Paris, Imagine Institute, Laboratory of Intestinal Immunity, INSERM UMR1163, Paris, France
e-mail: sacha.cording@inserm.fr; sofia.berrabah@inserm.fr

L. Lhermitte
Laboratory of Onco-Haematology, AP-HP, Hôpital Necker Enfants-Malades, Paris, France
e-mail: ludovic.lhermitte@aphp.fr

G. Malamut
Department of Gastroenterology, AP-HP. Centre-Université de Paris Hôpital Cochin, Paris, France

Université de Paris, Imagine Institute, Laboratory of Intestinal Immunity, INSERM UMR1163, Paris, France
e-mail: georgia.malamut@aphp.fr

N. Cerf-Bensussan (✉)
Laboratory of Intestinal Immunity, Université de Paris, INSERM UMR 1163 and Imagine Institute, Paris, France
e-mail: nadine.cerf-bensussan@inserm.fr

© Springer Nature Switzerland AG 2022
G. Malamut, N. Cerf-Bensussan (eds.), *Refractory Celiac Disease*,
https://doi.org/10.1007/978-3-030-90142-4_3

## The Long History of Intestinal Lymphoma in Celiac Disease

Hamilton Fairley and Mackie were likely the first to report on lymphoma in CeD, when they described in 1937 lymphomatous infiltration of mesenteric lymph nodes in four patients with clinical evidence of non-tropical sprue [1]. They suggested however that clinical symptoms and steatorrhea were secondary to lymphatic block-ade, a hypothesis which remained prevalent in several reports of lymphomas associ-ated with sprue-like disease that were published over the next 25 years. First suggestion that intestinal lymphoma is a complication of CeD was put forward in 1962 by Gough et al., who observed that the then called "small intestinal reticulo-sarcomas" were often preceded by CeD or idiopathic steatorrhea (a diagnosis retained when CeD had not be ascertained by histology and response to gluten-free-diet (GFD) [2]). Their hypothesis was confirmed in 1967 by Harris et al., who reported a series of 13 intestinal lymphomas in 202 adult patients with CeD or idiopathic steatorrhea, who had been followed-up in Birmingham between 1941 and 1965 [3]. These authors made two important observations. First a long period (mean 21 years) generally separated the initial diagnosis of CeD and the onset of lym-phoma. Second the incidence was perhaps less in patients treated by GFD. They therefore suggested the predisposing role of chronic inflammation and, conversely, possible protection by GFD [3]. Later follow-up of the "Birmingham cohort" until 1985, led Holmes et al. to suggest a 43-fold increase in the risk of lymphomas in CeD and to confirm the protective role of GFD [4]. Notably, no patient developed a lymphoma after 5 years on strict GFD. Since this historical study on a relatively small cohort, the incidence of lymphoma has been reappraised in much larger cohorts of CeD patients and the meta-analysis published in 2005 fortunately indi-cated an increase in relative risk that did not exceed three-fold [5]. Protection by the GFD, confirmed in these more recent studies and broadly used to treat CeD over the past 50 years, may perhaps contribute to this lesser incidence. Overall these data demonstrate that CeD predisposes to intestinal lymphoma. They support the view that lymphomagenesis is favored by the chronic autoimmune-like inflammation induced by gluten in CeD patients.

## The Intraepithelial Origin of Lymphoma Complicating Celiac Disease

Once the link with CeD was established, hot debate ensued on lymphoma cellular origin. The term of "reticulosarcoma" was first replaced by that of "malignant his-tiocytosis of the intestine", on the basis of morphological evidence suggestive of a monocyte-histiocyte lineage [6]. In 1985, the use of anti-CD3 and anti-CD7 anti-bodies and the demonstration of T cell receptor (TCR) γ rearrangements in three cases of CeD-associated lymphoma led Isaacson et al. to revise this view and to suggest a T cell lineage [7], a hypothesis supported by Salter et al. who showed CD3 and CD2 positivity in six additional cases [8]. The name of "enteropathy associated T lymphomas (EATL), almost immediately coined by O'Farelly et al. [9], has been retained in the present international classification of lymphomas [10].

Two observations next led to suggest the origin of EATL from intraepithelial lymphocytes (IEL). The first one, made by Isaacson et al., was the marked epitheliotropism of the tumoral cells [7]. The second one was the massive expansion of IEL in active CeD. This characteristic feature of CeD, first demonstrated by Ferguson and Murray [11], indeed suggested that IEL might escape regulation in active CeD and, as a consequence, give rise to EATL. Demonstration that most EATL stained with HML-1 [12], an antibody directed against the $\alpha_E\beta_7$ integrin (CD103) that is almost exclusively expressed by IEL in humans, provided the first clue to support this hypothesis [13, 14].

Definitive demonstration of the intraepithelial origin of EATL was provided by concordant observations indicating that, in many cases, overt lymphoma was preceded by a low-grade intraepithelial lymphoproliferation. Several reports summarized by Isaacson and Wright as early as in 1978 suggested that ulcerative jejunitis, a severe condition characterized by multiple large ulcers in the small intestine, could be associated but also precede CeD-associated lymphoma and may therefore be a premalignant condition. The authors noted that ulcerative lesions, although usually deprived of obviously neoplastic cells, were heavily infiltrated by mononuclear cells. This infiltrate was even defined as "pseudolymphoma" in a patient, who subsequently developed EATL (reviewed in [6]). In 1989, Alfsen et al. proposed the term of intraepithelial lymphoma to qualify the dense and diffuse small intestinal intraepithelial infiltration that they observed away from the neoplastic lesions in one case of EATL [15]. A parental relationship between the infiltrating IEL and the EATL was suggested by their common phenotype (CD3+ CD7+ HML-1+ but CD2− CD4− and CD8−) and by the detection of a TcRβ clonal rearrangement in biopsies sampled away from EATL. No comparison with the putative clonality of the EATL was however possible, preventing definitive conclusion [15]. Following this report, Wright et al. described one case of ulcerative jejunitis without EATL in which intense intraepithelial lymphocytosis was associated with the presence of a clonal TCRβ rearrangement. These authors further suggested that adult onset CeD might be an intraepithelial low-grade lymphoproliferation predisposing to EATL [16]. This hypothesis was discarded when later work showed that clonal intraepithelial lymphoproliferation was the appanage of rare but most severe complicated forms of CeD that were refractory to GFD (clonal RCD). The latter cases were often associated with ulcerative jejunitis and were at high risk to develop EATL [17–20].

One important next step was the Isolation of the "cytologically normal" IEL from the duodenal biopsies of patients with clonal RCD. It allowed to ascertain that these IEL carried the clonal TCRγ rearrangement detected in the biopsies [19] and to characterize their unusual phenotype [19]. In keeping with their reactivity with anti-CD3ε antibodies in tissue sections, clonal RCD IEL were shown to contain intracellular CD3ε. Yet, strikingly, they lacked surface CD3-TCR complexes and generally CD8 and thus differed from IEL from controls and uncomplicated active CeD that are mainly T cells (70–90% CD8+ TcRαβ+ and 15–30% TCRγδ). Filiation between clonal RCD IEL and EATL was definitively established by demonstrating the same clonal TCR rearrangement in the EATL as in the biopsies and in the clonal IEL that circulated in the blood 36 months before EATL onset [20].

As detailed below, clonal RCD has been now renamed type 2 RCD (RCD2) to stress the difference with other cases of RCD (classified as type 1 RCD) in which IEL are, as in active CeD, polyclonal T cells mainly CD8+ TCRαβ+ [21].

## Analysis of the Transition from Uncomplicated CeD to Type 1 and Type 2 Refractory CeD and EATL

Since the discovery of the causative role of gluten by W. Dicke in the 1950s [22], the only treatment of CeD remains a strict lifelong GFD. Studies led over the past 30 years have established how the human leucocyte antigens (HLA)-DQ2 or -DQ8 that confer the main genetic risk, can present undigested gluten peptides to intestinal CD4+ T cells and stimulate their production of cytokines, notably IL-2, IL-21 and IFNγ (reviewed in [23, 24]). Parallel studies have shown that another cytokine, interleukin 15(IL-15) is produced in excess during active CeD by stressed intestinal epithelial and *lamina propria* myeloid cells [25] and synergizes with cytokines released by gluten-specific CD4+ T cells to induce the expansion and activation of CD8+ TCRαβ+ IEL [26, 27]. The latter cells can then mount a cytolytic attack against epithelial cells that leads to the typical lesions of villous atrophy [28–30]. Although the mechanism underlying the excessive production of IL-15 in active CeD remains to be elucidated, this scenario has been authenticated in mouse models that combine intestinal overexpression of IL-15 and activation of CD4+ T cells by a dietary antigen [26, 27]. In one model combining transgenic expression of human HLA-DQ8 to promote gluten presentation to murine CD4+ T cells and that of IL-15 in intestinal epithelial and myeloid cells, epithelial recovery could be obtained by eliminating either CD8+ or CD4+ T cells or by withdrawing gluten, recapitulating the curative effect of GFD [27]. By preventing the activation of gluten-specific CD4+ T cells, GFD is thus sufficient to stop intestinal inflammation and to allow histological and clinical recovery. Although the curative effect of the GFD is observed in the vast majority of CeD patients, it is now clear that a small subset of patients may be or become refractory to GFD and remain with villous atrophy despite their strict adherence to this diet. True refractoriness to GFD is often difficult to establish. Indeed, histological response to GFD can be slow, notably in adults [31]. Moreover, inadvertent intake of gluten is frequent given the widespread presence of gluten in processed food. Overall, it is currently estimated that no more than 0.5% of CeD patients are truly refractory to GFD [32]. Such refractoriness can develop after an initial response to GFD or straight from diagnosis, notably when diagnosis is made late in life, likely after years of a pauci- or non-symptomatic form of CeD, pointing again to the aggravating role of long-lasting chronic inflammation [33, 34].

In CeD patients, who fail to respond to GFD, a first diagnosis to consider is EATL, notably if fever and recent wasting are present. Yet EATL revelation is often sudden due to intestinal obstruction or perforation requiring emergency surgery [35]. In the absence of EATL, two types of RCD have been individualized depending on the characteristics of IEL. As indicated above, type 2 RCD (RCD2) is defined by the presence of a clonal population of IEL which, in the vast majority of cases, do not express surface CD3-TCR complexes while containing intracellular CD3 and clonal DNA TCR rearrangements. This condition is associated in 60% of the cases with ulcerative jejunitis, which contributes to explain the severe malnutrition and profound hypoalbuminemia often observed in RCD2. The risk to develop an EATL is high, approximately 40% after 5 years [33, 34]. Even in the absence of EATL, the clonal cells display an invasive behavior. They are present along the small intestinal epithelium and they often disseminate to the gastric or colonic epithelium. They can also disseminate into *lamina propria*, into blood and eventually to other organs, notably liver, skin and lungs [33, 36, 37]. Yet, despite their dissemination, RCD2 cells differ from EATL cells as they remain small and do not divide actively as attested by their lack of positivity with anti-KI67 antibody [35]. Accordingly, they show very limited sensitivity to traditional chemotherapy. As compared to RCD2, RCD1 has usually a much milder clinical presentation. It is never associated with ulcerative jejunitis but collagenous sprue is frequent. As in controls and in uncomplicated CeD, IEL have a normal T cell phenotype and are mainly CD8+ TCRαβ+. In some cases, as in uncomplicated CeD on GFD, the proportion of TCRγδIEL (generally CD8−) can be increased above 25% (reviewed in [21]). The mechanism of resistance to GFD is not clearly defined in RCD1 but one plausible hypothesis is the onset of gluten-independent autoimmunity, a hypothesis supported by the increased frequency of extra-intestinal autoimmunity as compared to uncomplicated CeD (G. Malamut, unpublished observations). The onset of EATL, observed in some patients, is much less frequent than in RCD2. Thus, in a retrospective study of 37 cases of EATL diagnosed between 1992 and 2010 in four large hospitals in Paris, Malamut et al. observed that EATL complicated 20 cases of RCD2, two cases of RCD1 and 15 cases of CeD, which responded to GFD prior to lymphoma (n = 5) or during lymphoma treatment. Strikingly however, EATL prognosis was radically different depending on the underlying form of CeD: thus, survival at 5 years was almost 60% in EATL complicating RCD1 or GFD-responsive CeD but 0% in EATL complicating RCD2 [35].

## *Identification of the Intraepithelial Precursor(s) of RCD2 Lymphocytes from a Subset of Innate-like iCD3+ IEL* (Fig. 1)

Precise characterization of RCD2 IEL has benefited from their isolation and from the derivation of RCD2-IEL lines from duodenal biopsies. These studies have highlighted their dual T and NK cell features.

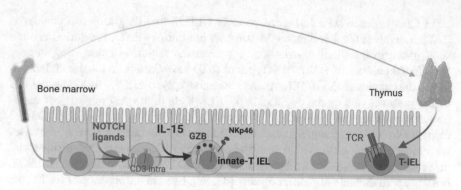

**Fig. 1** Differentiation of innate-like T-IEL according to [38]. In contrast to T-IEL, which undergo intrathymic differentiation before migrating into the gut, innate-like T IEL differentiate within the gut epithelium from hematopoietic/lymphoid precursors issued from the bone marrow. Thanks to the presence of NOTCH ligands in the gut epithelium, the latter cells can initiate T cell differentiation as attested by CD3 expression and presence of T cell receptor DNA rearrangements. Yet, T cell differentiation is switched off prematurely by IL-15. Indeed IL-15 produced by the gut epithelium, induces granzyme B (GZB), a protease that cleaves NOTCH into a peptide deprived of transcriptional activity. As a consequence, innate-like T- IEL cannot complete T cell differentiation and, by default, reverse to an NK fate characterized by acquisition of NK receptors (notably NKp46) and NK functions (Created with Biorender)

As indicated, in over 90% of cases, RCD2 IEL do not express surface CD3 (sCD3−) or TCR. They never express CD4, while CD8α is detected in only 30% of cases and sometimes variably in time ([19, 33, 37] and unpublished). RCD2 IEL possess however several hallmarks of T cells. First, they display intracellular expression of CD3ε and CD3γ [38] and probably of all CD3 chains (ε, γ, δ and ζ), as suggested by metabolic labeling of several RCD2 cell lines [39]. Second, as discussed above, DNA analysis show clonal TCR rearrangements. Strikingly, RCD2 IEL also share many features with NK cells. They display a broad spectrum of NK receptors at their surface. Some are shared with CD8+ T-IEL, notably NKG2D present in all human CD8+ T cells and CD94 that is upregulated in CD8+ T-IEL during active CeD [28–30, 40]. Others are more selectively expressed by RCD2 IEL. This is notably the case of NKp46, an activating NK receptor that is largely restricted to NK cells and to innate lymphoid cells [38]. In humans, NKp46 is also expressed by the small subset of TCRγδ Vδ1+ IEL that is present in the normal gut. Yet the latter cells disappear in active CeD during which they are durably replaced by a distinct subset of TCRγδ Vδ1+ IEL lacking NKp46 [41, 42]. Accordingly, most T-IEL in CeD do not express NKP46 [40] and NKP46 has emerged as an accurate diagnosis marker for RCD2 that can be detected in paraffin sections [43]. Alike NK cells but also CD8+ T-IEL, RCD2 IEL show strong dependency on IL-15 for their survival and activation. In the presence of IL-15, RCD2 IEL can notably produce IFNγ and exert strong NK-like cytotoxicity against enterocyte cell lines. Cytotoxicity of RCD2 IEL against enterocyte-lines was shown to depend on perforin and granzymes, to be facilitated by CD103-dependent adhesion to epithelial E-cadherin, and to be triggered upon engagement of the activating NKG2D receptor by MICA

(MHC class I polypeptide-related sequence A) [25, 29, 44]. Since IL-15 and the non-classical HLA class I molecule MICA are upregulated in enterocytes during RCD2 [25, 29], it is likely that RCD2 IEL can kill epithelial cells *in vivo*, and are thereby responsible for the severe epithelial lesions of villus atrophy and ulcerative jejunitis that accompany this condition.

The unusual but stereotypical phenotype of RCD2 IEL strongly suggested their origin from a common precursor present in the normal intestine. Given the massive expansion of CD8+ T-IEL which upregulate NK receptors and can exert NK-like activity in active CeD [28–30, 40, 45], it was first thought that RCD2 IEL derived from CD8+ TCRαβ+ IEL that had lost expression of their TCR. In depth characterization of the clonal TCR rearrangements in 28 cases of RCD failed however to reveal in frame rearrangements of both the α and β TCR, precluding their origin from TCRαβ+ IEL [38]. Moreover, in frame γ and δ TCR rearrangements were only present in eight cases (28%), demonstrating that, in the vast majority of patients, RCD2 IEL derived from lymphocytes that had initiated but not completed αβT cell differentiation [38]. The lack of surface TCR in RCD2 IEL even with in-frame γ and δ TCR rearrangements further suggested that the latter cells had not completed T cell maturation. It was therefore possible that RCD2 IEL rather derived from the small subset of sCD3-IEL that is present in the small intestine [46]. In keeping with this hypothesis, we observed that a fraction of the sCD3-IEL present in the normal gut co-expressed NK receptors, notably NKP46, with intracellular CD3ε and CD3 γ and also displayed polyclonal TCRγ and δ rearrangements [38]. Extending prior work [47], we next showed that a comparable subset of NKp46+ sCD3−iCD3+ lymphocytes could be differentiated *in vitro* by culturing human hematopoietic precursors in the presence of both NOTCH ligands and IL-15. According to its well-known role in T cell differentiation, activation of the NOTCH pathway licensed differentiation of lymphocytes that contained intracellular CD3ε and CD3γ and polyclonal TCRγ and δ rearrangements. In the presence of IL-15 however, T cell differentiation stopped prematurely, and T cell precursors were redirected to an NK cell fate attested by the acquisition of NKp46 and of NK effector functions. Mechanistically, IL-15 was shown to induce the protease Granzyme B, which cleaved the nuclear factor NOTCH1 into a transcriptionally inactive fragment, thereby shutting down the transcriptional program that is indispensable to achieve complete T cell differentiation [38] (Fig. 1). This *in vitro* scenario was validated by *in vivo* studies in mice, which also display a small subset of sCD3-IEL containing intracellular CD3 and TCR rearrangements [48–50]. Hematopoietic precursors cells isolated from bone marrow and transferred into recipient mice migrated into the intestine where they gave rise to sCD3-IEL containing intracellular CD3γ through a mechanism that required NOTCH, IL-15 and granzyme B. Transfer into thymectomized mice allowed to eliminate any thymic contribution [38]. Altogether, our studies indicate that besides T-IEL that seed the intestine after intrathymic differentiation, some hematopoietic precursors can migrate directly into the gut epithelium and give rise locally to a small but heterogenous population of innate lymphoid cells. Since NOTCH ligands are expressed in the gut epithelium [51], hematopoietic precursors that reach the intestine may initiate T cell differentiation, which is prematurely stopped by IL-15. This cytokine, perhaps together with other cytokines present in the gut environment, can then stimulate the differentiation of sCD3-IEL into innate effector lymphoid cells that produce IFNγ or exert NK-like cytotoxicity. IL-15 can also promote their local survival [38] (Fig. 1).

While in most patients, RCD2 arise from a small subset of iCD3+ innate-like lymphoid cells present in the normal intestine, this rule is not absolute. Thus, we and others have observed rare cases of RCD2 IEL with cell surface expression of a clonal TCRγδ and in one case, of a clonal TCRαβ [37, 43, 52]. Conversely, we have also observed two cases displaying NK receptors but lacking intracellular CD3 and TCR rearrangement (unpublished data). The latter examples indicate that malignant transformation is not strictly restricted to iCD3+ innate-like IEL. Yet, the selective development of RCD2 from the latter small subset of IEL is puzzling. One may speculate that TCR rearrangement introduces DNA instability that is absent in the iCD3− subset of IEL that resemble NK cells or type 1 innate lymphoid cells. Conversely, expression of a functional TCR may safeguard T cells against transformation, perhaps by providing signals that limit T cell expansion or induce apoptosis.

## JAK1-STAT3 Mutations in RCD2 Link Chronic Inflammation and Lymphomagenesis (Fig. 2)

As stressed above, innate iCD3+ IEL form a very tiny fraction of IEL in the normal intestine and their frequency is even less in active CeD due to the massive expansion of T-IEL. One important characteristic of RCD2 IEL is their high responsiveness to IL-15. Accordingly, *in vitro* survival and expansion of RCD2 IEL require much lesser concentrations of IL-15 than CD8+ T-IEL [25, 53]. This property has been very useful to derive RCD2 lines from duodenal biopsies. It also suggested that RCD2 IEL might have acquired somatic mutations that foster their response to IL-15 and enable them to outgrow residual normal T-IEL in the CeD intestine. This hypothesis has been substantiated by our recent genomic studies.

A comprehensive catalogue of the somatic genetic events associated with malignant transformation was first established in pure populations of RCD2 cells using whole exome sequencing (WES), chromosomal genomic hybridization (CGH) and RNAseq [37]. The small number of RCD2 IEL that can be isolated from biopsies precluded the use of these unbiased approaches. We therefore used IL-15-dependent RCD2 cell lines derived from biopsies and, in two patients with a large number of circulating RCD2 cells, CD103+sCD3−RCD2 cells FACS-sorted from fresh blood. This analysis, possible in 10 patients, revealed a complex mutational landscape with a mean of 70 potentially oncogenic somatic mutations (39–102) and numerous chromosomal abnormalities. Strikingly all patients showed mutations predicted to activate the JAK1-STAT3 pathway and nine had deleterious mutations, mainly copy number variations, in either A20/TNFAIP3, a potent negative regulator of NF-kB or in its partner TNIP3. Recurrent mutations were also found in several epigenetic

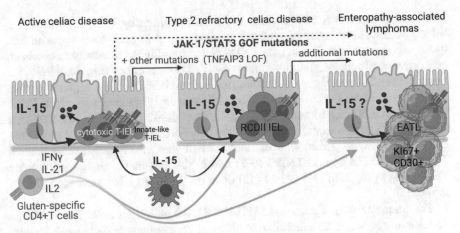

**Fig. 2** Hypothetical scheme depicting celiac disease associated lymphomagenesis. In CeD, lymphoma arise from IEL and notably from innate-like T IEL. The latter cells are sparse in uncomplicated active CeD in which they are outnumbered by the massive expansion of CD8+ TcRαβ+ IEL that is driven by the cooperative interactions between cytokines released by gluten-specific CD4+ T cells and IL-15 produced by enterocytes and by lamina propria myeloid cells. In type 2 refractory CeD (RCD2), due to the acquisition of somatic gain of function (GOF) mutations in the JAK1-STAT3 pathway, a clone of innate-like T IEL can compete very efficiently for the same cocktail of cytokines and progressively outcompete normal T-IEL, a process sustained by the acquisition of additional mutations, notably in *TNFAIP3*, which enhances activation of the NF-KB pathway, and in epigenetic regulators (see text) that promote genome instability and further transformation. Accumulation of mutations can ultimately lead to transformation into EATL. Direct transformation from active CeD into EATL is however possible in a subset of patients without any evidence of RCD2. As in EATL complicating RCD2, the oncogenetic landscape is dominated by GOF mutations in the JAK-STAT3 pathway pointing to the key role of the cytokine environment in driving lymphomagenesis. It is however likely that at the stage of EATL, malignant cells can proliferate and invade tissues largely independently of inflammatory cytokine (Created with Biorender)

modifiers known to control oncogenesis, notably KMT2D and TET2. The considerable overlap observed in one patient between the mutational profile of the biopsy-derived RCD2 line and of RCD2 cells isolated from fresh blood indicated that most mutations present in the biopsy-derived cell line had been acquired prior to culture. This was notably the case of the *JAK1* and *TNFAIP3* mutations. Interestingly, several mutations were detected only in RCD2 cells isolated from fresh blood pointing-out to intra-tumor heterogeneity that may have perhaps promoted dissemination of RCD2 cells outside the gut [37].

In order to confirm and to extend these results to a larger cohort of 50 RCD2 cases, duodenal biopsies were analyzed by targeted next generation sequencing. This method can only detect mutations in the panel of genes selected for study but is more sensitive than WES to identify somatic events in tissues with limited tumor infiltration. Each biopsy was studied by two panels: one covered the exons of 104 genes in which pathogenic mutations associated with T cell malignancies have been annotated in the Cosmic data base and or previously reported. The second panel encompassed 69 genes of the first panel in which mutations were detected and 22 additional genes in which mutations had been identified by WES in pure RCD2 cells. Overall, the number of mutated genes detected in each biopsy (mean 3.9; 0–10) was much lower than in pure RCD2 cells, stressing the difficulty to obtain an exhaustive catalogue of mutations and notably of copy number variations in RCD2 biopsies [37]. Despite these limitations, this analysis confirmed the high recurrence of mutations in JAK1 (48%) and STAT3 (38%) as well as in the negative JAK-STAT regulators SOCS1 (12%) and SOCS3 (8%). Overall, 43 out of 50 (86%) patients showed at least one somatic alteration of the JAK1-STAT3 axis. It was also possible to also confirm the recurrence of mutations in the NF-κB negative regulators TNFAIP3/A20 (13%) and TNIP3 (9%) and in the epigenetic regulators, notably TET2 (30%) [54], KMT2D (22%) [55] or in the X-linked RNA helicase DDX3X [56] (20%).

The demonstration of recurrent JAK1 and STAT3 mutations in RCD2 provides a decisive link between chronic inflammation and lymphomagenesis in CeD. Indeed, JAK1 is one of four Janus kinases that, upon binding of several inflammatory cytokines, can phosphorylate STAT3, allowing its dimerization and nuclear translocation and, as a consequence, induction of a broad transcriptional program that participates in activation, differentiation, survival and proliferation of many lymphocytes subsets [57, 58]. In RCD2, STAT3 mutations were predominantly found in the regulatory SH2 domain with notably mutations in p.661 that are known to enhance STAT3 dimerization and activation [59]. Comparable STAT3 mutations have been described in several cancers and notably in large granular lymphocyte leukemias, which are thought to be favored by IL-15 [60]. Even more strikingly, almost all JAK1 mutations clustered at the p.1097 position in the C-terminal JH1-kinase domain, a highly conserved position, and the site of interaction of the JAK1 negative regulator SOCS1 [61].

Several cytokines that activate the JAK-STAT pathway are produced in active CeD, including IFNγ, IL-2, IL-6, IL-21 and IL-15 [25, 62, 63]. While IL-21 and IL-6 are strong inducers of the JAK-1-STAT3 cascade, IFNγ rather induces JAK1-STAT1 while IL-2 and IL-15 preferentially induce JAK3-STAT5 signaling. Importantly, functional studies performed in RCD2 IEL lines indicate that, in most cases, these mutations do not result in constitutive STAT3 activation. In contrast, they license and sustain activation of the JAK1-STAT3 cascade in response to IL-15. Accordingly, STAT3 phosphorylation was strongly induced in RCD2 IEL lines by very low concentrations of IL-15, which had no effect on cell lines derived from normal T-IEL [37, 38]. It is tempting to suggest that simultaneous activation of JAK3-STAT5 and JAK1-STAT3 by IL-15 endows RCD2 IEL with a selective advantage to outcompete normal T cells in the inflamed CeD intestine. The effect of IFNγ, IL-2, IL-6 and IL-21 on RCD2 cell lines was not tested. Yet, it is likely that the latter cytokines may also foster activation and or expansion of RCD2 cells. Overall, these data explain how cytokines produced in the inflamed gut can synergize with JAK1 and STAT3 GOF mutations to drive the emergence of RCD2, and more generally to drive CeD-associated lymphomagenesis as further discussed below (Fig. 2).

Additional mutations may also stimulate activation and expansion of RCD2 IEL in the inflamed CeD gut. This is notably the case of recurrent deletion, frameshift or stop-gain mutations in TNFAIP3/A20 or in its partner TNIP3. If the role of TNIP3 is not yet well delineated [64], TNFAIP3/A20 is a potent negative regulator of NF-κB. Inactivating mutations are frequent in lymphomas where they can potentiate survival in response to inflammatory signals [65]. Constitutive monoallelic inactivating mutation in TNFAIP3/A20 can also cause severe intestinal inflammation (reviewed in [66]). Moreover NF-κB and STAT3 may cooperate to promote protumorogenic gene expression [67]. In keeping with a possible contribution of inactivating TNFAIP/3A20 mutations to oncogenesis, constitutive activation of NF-kB or its enhanced activation by TNFα was observed in RCD2 lines carrying mutations in TNFAIP3/A20. The secretion of TNFα described in gluten-sensitized CD4+ T cells [68] as well as in T-IEL from CeD patients [69] may therefore foster expansion or activation of RCD2 cells. An autocrine loop involving NF-kB-induced production of STAT3 activating cytokines by RCD2 cells, as described in some B cell lymphomas [70], is also possible.

In keeping with these results, a recent study that sequenced 465 genes associated with cancer in the biopsies of 11 patients classified as RCD2 showed an overlapping spectrum of mutations including the JAK1p1097 hot spot, mutations in STAT3 SH2, and predicted LOF mutations in *TNFAIP3, TET2, KMT2D*. Whether all patients had RCD2 is however not completely sure. Thus, it was unclear if they all had CeD; only eight had the typical sCD3−iCD3+ phenotype ascertained by FACS and one case had a very unusual CD4+ phenotype [71].

## *EATL Complicating RCD2 or Occurring* De Novo *in Celiac Disease or RCD1 Share a Mutational Landscape Dominated by JAK1 and STAT3 Mutations* (Fig. 2)

Data above lead to propose that mutations activating the JAK1- STAT3 and, in some cases, the NF-κB pathways, act in concert with cytokines released in the inflammatory CeD intestine to stimulate the clonal expansion of malignant RCD2 cells, their autonomous production of cytokines and their cytotoxicity against epithelial cells, overall creating a vicious circle that promotes genomic instability, accumulation of genetic aberrations and ultimately transformation into EATL (Fig. 2). This scenario is supported by the mutational landscape observed in EATL complicating RCD2 (RCD2-EATL) [37]. Using the same targeted approach as for RCD2, we observed that JAK1, STAT3 and TNFAIP3/A20 mutations were never lost during progression to EATL. In contrast, a spectrum of additional pathogenic mutations was detected in EATL compared to autologous RCD2 sampled before EATL. The variable frequency of pathogenic variants in both RCD2 and EATL biopsies pointed out to intratumor heterogeneity with coexistence of different subclones containing diverse combinations of mutations, some of which might be more particularly oncogenic [37]. This may notably be the case for combinations of mutations in JAK1 and STAT3. Indeed, previous work using a clonogenic *in vitro* assay has shown how mutations in JAK1p1097 and STAT3p661 can synergize to promote transformation in the presence of IL-6 [72]. In keeping with a possible predictive value of the latter combination, its detection in RCD2 biopsies before EATL development was associated with increased risk of EATL. The lack of statistically significant difference, perhaps due to the relatively small size of the cohort, precludes however any definitive conclusion [37].

As indicated, EATL can complicate RCD2 but may also develop *de novo* in patients with RCD1 or with active CeD that responds to GFD when EATL has been treated [35]. The much less pejorative prognosis of *de novo* EATL than of RCD2-EATL (60% versus 0% survival at 5 years) suggested that distinctive oncogenic events might underlie these two entities. Arguing against this hypothesis, targeted next generation sequencing showed comparable mutational landscapes and comparable numbers of mutations in the 11 cases of RCD2-EATL and in the eight cases of *de novo* EATL that were studied simultaneously (Fig. 2). One significant difference was the constant presence of the hot spot JAK1p1097 mutation in *de novo* EATL versus 55% in RCD2-EATL but it remains unclear why it should lead to a distinct prognosis. A second notable difference was the lack of detectable mutation in TNFAIP3/A20 in *de novo* EATL [37]. Yet, the latter difference will need confirmation as the number of *de novo* EATL was small and copy number variations in *TNFAIP3* might have been missed. Therefore, it seems difficult to ascribe the drastic difference in prognosis to distinct mutational profiles. An alternative and more plausible hypothesis is that RCD2 provides a vast reservoir of clonal malignant cells which, due to their very low proliferative rate, are not sensible to the chemotherapy regimen used to treat EATL. They can therefore persist, undergo further transformation and thereby cause EATL relapse.

Overall our data are consistent with a driving role of JAKp1097-STAT3-SH2 GOF mutations in CeD-associated lymphomagenesis, whether EATL develops in one step or in two-steps after a first phase of RCD2. In keeping with this conclusion, JAK1p1097 and GOF STAT3-SH2 mutations were also detected in five out of the eight EATL (denominated EATLI according to the previous international classification of lymphomas) analyzed by Roberti et al. [73]. As these authors performed WES on formalin-fixed paraffin-embedded tissues, it is even not excluded that the three remaining cases were false negative. Of note, mutations in the JAK-STAT pathway are frequent in intestinal T lymphoproliferations, pointing to a common mechanism whereby mutations interact with inflammatory cytokines to drive intestinal lymphomagenesis. The nature of the mutations can however vary. STAT3-JAK2 fusion proteins and GOF mutations in STAT3-SH2 have been recurrently detected in indolent T cell lymphoproliferative disorders, a generally moderately aggressive clonal T cell disorder [74, 75]. In contrast, GOF mutations in *JAK3* or *STAT5B* are a hallmark of monomorphic epitheliotropic intestinal T-cell lymphomas (MEITL), a second form of very aggressive intestinal lymphoma that is not associated with CeD but is also thought to arise from IEL, notably TCRγδ IEL [73, 76]. At odd with these results, Moffit et al. have reported high occurrence of loss-of-function (LOF) SETD2 mutations, and of JAK3 and STAT5B GOF mutations in

EATL [77]. Yet, it is likely that some lymphomas classified as EATL might have been in fact MEITL. Thus, CeD was present in only 84% of EATL but also, unexpectedly in 16% cases classified as MEITL, which are not associated with CeD, according to WHO guidelines. Moreover, SETD2 LOF mutations have also been predominantly associated with MEITL by Roberti et al. [73]. If *STAT3* GOF mutations are commonly observed in many lymphoproliferative disorders in and outside the gut, this is not the case of the JAK1p1097 mutations which, besides RCD2 and EATL, have been almost exclusively observed in a small subset of anaplastic ALK-negative lymphomas, notably in a subset of those developing around breast implants that are also driven by chronic inflammation [72, 78]. The JAK1p1097 mutations may thus represent an interesting diagnosis marker for RCD2 and EATL together as a signature for cytokine-driven lymphomagenesis.

## Lessons for Therapy in RCD2

Deciphering the mechanisms underlying CeD-associated lymphomagenesis has entirely validated observations first made over 50 years ago, which pointed to the protective role of GFD. It is now clear that, by switching off excessive production of inflammatory cytokines, GFD can prevent the selection of transformed lymphocytes. If GFD is no more sufficient at the stage of RCD2 and EATL, it does remain indispensable to reduce as drastically as possible the inflammatory milieu, which fosters tumor progression. In this regard, it is noticeable that some RCD2 patients in clinical and histological remission after treatment by steroids may remain clinically silent several years on GFD alone despite the persistence of the clonal intracpithelial RCD2 IEL cells ([33] and unpublished observations). Yet, several of them have progressed toward EATL, stressing the need to delineate complementary therapeutic strategies.

Given their malignant character, it would ideally be best to eradicate RCD2 cells. This is however not simple. As indicated, RCD2 cells have low proliferative rate and are therefore refractory to classical aggressive chemotherapies. Mulder and colleagues have proposed to use the deoxyadenosine analogue cladribrine (2-chlorodeoxyadenosine) [79]. Due to the substitution of a chlorine atom for the hydrogen atom at the 2-position of the purine ring, cladribine is resistant to adenosine-desaminase and can be incorporated into DNA but also induce cell death in non-replicative cells [80]. Accordingly, monotherapy by cladribine could decrease the number of RCD2 IEL and, in a subset of patients induce histological remission, which correlated with a lesser transformation into EATL. The risk of EATL however persisted. Moreover, EATL incidence was high in patients without histological recovery even if the number of RCD2 IEL had decreased [81] and EATL onset occurred rapidly in several patients [33]. It is not excluded that the strong and durable CD4+ lymphopenia induced by cladribine might promote EATL development. As an alternative to chemotherapy, it has been proposed to destroy malignant RCD2 cells by targeting a membrane antigen expressed by RCD2 IEL. Following treatment by the anti-CD52 antibody Alentezumab, Vivas et al. observed clinical and histological remission in one patient [82]. Yet, due to the broad expression of CD52 on all mature lymphocytes, dendritic cells and monocytes, this treatment induces very severe immunosuppression exposing to life-threatening infections and perhaps promoting EATL onset, which occurred rapidly in a second patient treated by anti-CD52 antibody [33]. It seems therefore indispensable to identify targets that could avoid such broad lymphocyte deletion. In contrast to EATL, RCD2 IEL do not express CD30, precluding the use of Brentuximab [37]. One interesting target antigen introduced above is NKp46, which has very limited tissue expression. The paucity of CD16-expressing NK cells and macrophages in intestinal tissue suggests that antibody-dependent cell mediated cytotoxicity will fail to efficiently deplete RCD2 IEL. To circumvent this difficulty, an NKp46 antibody that can be internalized has been coupled with the cytotoxic drug pyrrolobenzodiazepine. This antibody could efficiently kill freshly isolated RCD2 IEL *in vitro* [83]. Demonstration of its clinical efficacy is however pending. An alternative option in the future may be to design CAR-T cells targeting NKp46. Several limitations can however be anticipated when targeting NKp46. Expression of NKp46 at the surface of RCD2 IEL can be weak and in some cases, NKp46 remains intracellular. In addition, NKp46 will also deplete NK cells and it cannot be excluded that this may impair host anti-tumor responses. Identification of other membrane antigens with restricted distribution might be useful.

Instead of targeting RCD2 cells, Murray and colleagues have rather advocated to reduce small intestinal inflammation by using oral corticoids under the form of open-capsule budesonide. They reported significant clinical and histological improvement in 13 RCD2 patients classified as RCD2 [84], a result confirmed in a larger cohort of patients followed up in Paris (Khater et al. in preparation). Budesonide may not only decrease production of inflammatory cytokines but also exert a direct inhibitory effect on RCD2 IEL. Thus, *in vitro* addition of budesonide to IL-15-dependent RCD2 cell lines reduced their proliferation and increased their apoptosis [37]. Some patients can however become dependent or refractory to budesonide. Moreover, retrospective analysis indicates that budesonide alone does not reduce the risk of progression toward EATL (Khater et al. in preparation).

Another option to break the vicious circle that link intestinal inflammation and outgrowth of RCD2 cells might be to block the interplay between IL-15 and the JAK1 and or STAT3 GOF mutations. Following evidence that the human anti-IL-15 antibody AMG714 blocked the anti-apoptotic and pro-proliferative effects of soluble IL-15 on RCD2 IEL lines *in vitro* [53], this antibody used in a recent clinical trial. Unfortunately, a three month-treatment had no effect on the number of RCD2 IEL and only marginally improved histology and clinical symptoms. Interpretation of these results is not completely straightforward. First, it is possible that AMG714 did not efficiently block IL-15 *in vivo*. Thus, frequency of peripheral NK cells, which are strongly dependent on IL-15, remained unchanged during treatment. Second, a positive effect of AMG714 might have been blurred by budesonide received by several patients before or during the trial [85]. Conversely, it is possible that blocking IL-15 might have negative effects by impairing putative anti-tumor responses. There is indeed multiple experimental and, since recently, some clinical evidence for the importance of IL-15 in sustaining NK or CD8-mediated anti-tumor responses [86]. The difficulty to monitor IL-15 concentrations further complicates definitive conclusions. An alternative option might be to block the JAK-STAT pathway and inhibit both RCD2 cell growth and local inflammation. *In vitro*, JAK3 or JAK1 inhibitors can act on IL-15-dependent RCD2 lines, inhibiting STAT5 or STAT3 phosphorylation respectively and, as a consequence inhibiting their proliferation and or inducing their apoptosis [37, 38, 53]. Of note, these drugs inhibited also strongly the growth and survival of cell lines derived from normal residual CD4+ and CD8+ T cells in RCD2 biopsies. This finding is not surprising given the dependence of the latter cell lines on IL-15 in the chosen experimental setting but, again, it raises concern on the risk to inhibit a putative anti-tumor response. Whether switching off the vicious inflammatory circle that promotes CeD- associated lymphomagenesis may outweigh the risk of impaired tumor surveillance therefore remains an open question. Pleading in favor of a beneficial role of JAK inhibitors is the recent observation that oncogenic activation STAT3 can drive autonomous PDL1 expression in natural/killer lymphomas [87]. More definitive answer may come soon from an on-going trial using the pan-JAK inhibitor Tofacinitib [88].

Given the frequency of mutations in NF-κB regulators in RCD2, a complementary treatment to JAK inhibitors might be the use of NF-κB inhibitors such as bortezomib, a drug approved for the treatment of multiple myeloma. Interestingly, this drug impaired the growth and induced the apoptosis of RCD2 cell lines without affecting that of normal T cell lines [37]. In keeping with previous observations in myeloma cells, this effect was accompanied by decreased STAT3 phosphorylation in RCD2 lines. In myeloma cells, bortezomib is thought to act by blocking NF-κB-induction of STAT3-activating cytokines (e.g. IL-6) [70]. Surprisingly however, inhibition of STAT3 phosphorylation was observed in RCD2 cell lines whether or not they displayed constitutive NF-κB activation. The rationale to use bortezomib alone or in combination with JAK inhibitors in RCD2 thus remains fragile.

Overall, dissecting the mutational landscape of RCD2 IEL has opened the way to personalized therapy that may, depending on the case, target JAK-STAT and or NF-κB as well perhaps as some mutated epigenetic modifiers. Yet, information is missing on a possible anti-tumor response that may be instrumental to contain RCD2 but inhibited by several of the drugs targeting the mutations. In addition, past experience in other cancers have shown how subclones carrying additional mutations may be selected by targeted treatments. This leads to consider other additional and possibly complementary therapeutic strategies.

One important option, initially advocated by Tack et al. is autologous stem cell transplantation (ASCT) following intensive chemotherapy and conditioning by fludarabine (a purine analogue acting similarly as cladribine) and melphalan [89]. In patients younger than 70 years who had failed to respond to cladribine, this treatment reduced very significantly the risk to develop EATL, which is very high in this subgroup of patients [81]. This strategy has also been successfully applied in a distinct cohort of RCD2 patients refractory to corticoids, who were followed up in Paris. Although rapid onset of EATL was observed during intensive chemotherapy in two patients, long term outcome in the small number of severely sick patients who underwent ASCT seems excellent. Despite rapid clinical and histological improvement, persistence of a very high frequency of RCD2 IEL following ASCT was initially worrying. Yet, strikingly, in all treated patients, the number of RCD2 IEL decreased slowly but steadily over the years with no further onset of EATL (unpublished observations). The mechanism by which ASCT may enable progressive elimination of RCD2 cells remains unknown. Resetting intestinal homeostasis may prevent the production of cytokines indispensable for their growth. Development of an anti-tumor response is however also possible. This possibility remains to be explored as it may open the path to vaccination in the future.

## Conclusion and Perspectives

Recent work has established how gluten-induced chronic inflammation can drive the clonal selection of innate-like T lymphocytes carrying mutations that enhance their responses to cytokines, ultimately leading to their transformation into lymphomas. This scenario is strongly reminiscent of that described since many years in extranodal mucosa-associated lymphoid tissue (MALT) B lymphomas in which cooperation between genetic abnormalities and chronic inflammation drive lymphomagenesis. This is notably the case of MALT lymphomas induced by *Helicobacter pylori* in the stomach [90] or of alpha chain immunoproliferative disease of the small intestine that has been associated with inappropriate responses to *Campylobacter jejuni*. In both situations, progression to overt lymphomas can be blocked at an early stage using antibiotics in order to switch off chronic immune stimulation and inflammation. Overall, it is likely that intestinal lymphomagenesis is most often driven by dysregulated chronic immune reactions that can develop in the highly exposed gut environment. Evidence of diverse possible causes of chronic inflammation in small intestinal CD4+ T cell indolent lymphomas, supports this view [91]. Along the same line, it is tempting to establish a parallel between the somatic JAK1/STAT3 GOF mutations driving CeD-associated lymphomagenesis and the constitutive mutations enhancing the JAK1/STAT3 pathway that are found in a substantial subset of patients with non-celiac forms of autoimmune enteropathies where they lead to uncontrolled activation of effector T cells (reviewed in [66]. Overall these findings provide a novel example of the overlap between the mechanisms that underlie autoimmunity and lymphocyte transformation and stress the need of a strict control of the JAK1-STAT3 pathway in order to maintain intestinal homeostasis.

In conclusion, the mechanisms underlying CeD-associated lymphomagenesis are now well delineated. Yet, much work remains ahead to define how to translate these findings into pertinent therapeutic strategies. It will notably be very important to define whether anti-tumor responses may develop in RCD2 and EATL and if so, to delineate the optimal therapeutic strategy that may neutralize the malignant cells while preserving or enhancing these protective immune responses.

**Grant Support** Work related to this chapter has been supported by institutional grants from INSERM and Université de Paris and by grants from ANR (Nr18-CE14–0005), Foundation ARC-Recherche Clinique (PGA1 RF20180206809), Foundation Princesse Grace and Association Française Des Intolérants au Gluten (AFDIAG). Institut Imagine is supported by Agence Nationale de la Recherche as part of the "Investment for the Future" program (ANR-10-IAHU-01).

# References

1. Fairley NH, Mackie FP. Clinical and biochemical syndrome in lymphadenoma. BMJ. 1937;1:375–404.
2. Gough KR, Read AE, Naish JM. Intestinal reticulosis as a complication of idiopathic steatorrhoea. Gut. 1962;3:232–9.
3. Harris OD, Cooke WT, Thompson H, et al. Malignancy in adult coeliac disease and idiopathic steatorrhoea. Am J Med. 1967;42:899–912.
4. Holmes GK, Prior P, Lane MR, et al. Malignancy in coeliac disease--effect of a gluten free diet. Gut. 1989;30:333–8.
5. Catassi C, Bearzi I, Holmes GKT. Association of celiac disease and intestinal lymphomas and other cancers. Gastroenterology. 2005;128:S79–86.
6. Isaacson P, Wright DH. Malignant histiocytosis of the intestine. Hum Pathol. 1978;9:661–77.
7. Isaacson PG, Spencer J, Connolly CE, et al. Malignant histiocytosis of the intestine: a t-cell lymphoma. Lancet. 1985;326:688–91.
8. Salter DM, Krajewski AS, Dewar AE. Immunophenotype analysis of malignant histiocytosis of the intestine. J Clin Pathol. 1986;39:8–15.
9. O'Farrelly C, Feighery C, O'Briain DS, et al. Humoral response to wheat protein in patients with coeliac disease and enteropathy associated T cell lymphoma. BMJ. 1986;293:908–10.
10. Swerdlow SH, Campo E, Pileri SA, et al. The 2016 revision of the World Health Organization classification of lymphoid neoplasms. Blood. 2016;127:2375–90.
11. Ferguson A, Murray D. Quantitation of intraepithelial lymphocytes in human jejunum. Gut. 1971;12:988–94.
12. Spencer J, Cerf-Bensussan N, Jarry A, et al. Enteropathy-associated T cell lymphoma (malignant histiocytosis of the intestine) is recognized by a monoclonal antibody (HML-1) that defines a membrane molecule on human mucosal lymphocytes. Am J Pathol. 1988;132:1–5.
13. Cerf-Bensussan N, Jarry A, Brousse N, et al. A monoclonal antibody (HML-1) defining a novel membrane molecule present on human intestinal lymphocytes. Eur J Immunol. 1987;17:1279–85.
14. Cerf-Bensussan N, Begue B, Gagnon J, et al. The human intraepithelial lymphocyte marker HML-1 is an integrin consisting of a beta 7 subunit associated with a distinctive alpha chain. Eur J Immunol. 1992;22:273–277 and 885.
15. Cecilie Alfsen G, Beiske K, Bell H, et al. Low-grade intestinal lymphoma of intraepithelial T lymphocyties with concomitant enteropathy-associated T cell lymphoma: case report suggesting a possible histogenetic relationship. Hum Pathol. 1989;20:909–13.
16. Wright DH, Jones DB, Clark H, et al. Is adult-onset coeliac disease due to a low-grade lymphoma of intraepithelial T lymphocytes? Lancet. 1991;337:1373–4.
17. Carbonnel F, Grollet-Bioul L, Brouet JC, et al. Are complicated forms of celiac disease cryptic T-cell lymphomas? Blood. 1998;92:3879–86.

18. Bagdi E, Diss TC, Munson P, et al. Mucosal intra-epithelial lymphocytes in enteropathy-associated T-cell lymphoma, ulcerative jejunitis, and refractory celiac disease constitute a neoplastic population. Blood. 1999;94:260–4.

19. Cellier C, Patey N, Mauvieux L, et al. Abnormal intestinal intraepithelial lymphocytes in refractory sprue. Gastroenterology. 1998;114:471–81.

20. Cellier C, Delabesse E, Helmer C, et al. Refractory sprue, coeliac disease, and enteropathy-associated T-cell lymphoma. French coeliac disease study group [see comments]. Lancet. 2000;356:203–8.

21. Malamut G, Cording S, Cerf-Bensussan N. Recent advances in celiac disease and refractory celiac disease. F1000Res. 2019;8:969.

22. Van de Kamer JH, Weijers HA, Dicke WK. Coeliac disease V. Some experiments on the cause of the harmful effect of wheat gliadin. Acta Paediatr Scand. 1953;42:223–31.

23. Jabri B, Sollid LM. Tissue-mediated control of immunopathology in coeliac disease. Nat Rev Immunol. 2009;9:858–70.

24. Meresse B, Malamut G, Cerf-Bensussan N. Celiac disease: an immunological jigsaw. Immunity. 2012;36:907–19.

25. Mention J-J, Ahmed M Ben, Bègue B, et al. Interleukin 15: a key to disrupted intraepithelial lymphocyte homeostasis and lymphomagenesis in celiac disease. Gastroenterology. 2003;125:730–45.

26. Korneychuk N, Ramiro-Puig E, Ettersperger J, et al. Interleukin 15 and CD4(+) T cells cooperate to promote small intestinal enteropathy in response to dietary antigen. Gastroenterology. 2014;146:1017–27.

27. Abadie V, Kim SM, Lejeune T, et al. IL-15, gluten and HLA-DQ8 drive tissue destruction in coeliac disease. Nature. 2020;578:600–4.

28. Meresse B, Chen Z, Ciszewski C, et al. Coordinated induction by IL15 of a TCR-independent NKG2D signaling pathway converts CTL into lymphokine-activated killer cells in celiac disease. Immunity. 2004;21:357–66.

29. Hue S, Mention JJ, Monteiro RC, et al. A direct role for NKG2D/MICA interaction in villous atrophy during celiac disease. Immunity. 2004;21:367–77.

30. Meresse B, Curran SA, Ciszewski C, et al. Reprogramming of CTLs into natural killer-like cells in celiac disease. J Exp Med. 2006;203:1343–55.

31. Wahab PJ, Meijer JWR, Mulder CJJ. Histologic follow-up of people with celiac disease on a gluten-free diet. Am J Clin Pathol. 2002;118:459–63.

32. Rowinski SA, Christensen E. Epidemiologic and therapeutic aspects of refractory coeliac disease - a systematic review. Dan Med J. 2016;63:A5307.

33. Malamut G, Afchain P, Verkarre V, et al. Presentation and long-term follow-up of refractory celiac disease: comparison of type I with type II. Gastroenterology. 2009;136:81–90.

34. Rubio–Tapia A, Kelly DG, Lahr BD, et al. Clinical staging and survival in refractory celiac disease: a single center experience. Gastroenterology. 2009;136:99–107.

35. Malamut G, Chandesris O, Verkarre V, et al. Enteropathy associated T cell lymphoma in celiac disease: a large retrospective study. Dig Liver Dis. 2013;45:377–84.

36. Verkarre V, Asnafi V, Lecomte T, et al. Refractory coeliac sprue is a diffuse gastrointestinal disease. Gut. 2003;52:205–11.

37. Cording S, Lhermitte L, Malamut G, Berrabah S, Trinquand A, Guegan N, Villarese P, Kaltenbach S, Meresse B, Khater S, Dussiot M, Bras M, Cheminant M, Tesson B, Bole-Feysot C, Bruneau J, Molina TJ, Sibon D, Macintyre E, Hermine O, Cellier C, Asnafi V, Cerf-Bensussan N; CELAC Network. Oncogenetic landscape of lymphomagenesis in coeliac disease. Gut. 2021. doi: https://doi.org/10.1136/gutjnl-2020-322935. Online ahead of print. PMID: 33579790.

38. Ettersperger J, Montcuquet N, Malamut G, et al. Interleukin-15-dependent T-cell-like innate intraepithelial lymphocytes develop in the intestine and transform into lymphomas in celiac disease. Immunity. 2016;45:610–25.

39. Tjon JM, Verbeek WH, Kooy-Winkelaar YM, et al. Defective synthesis or association of T-cell receptor chains underlies loss of surface T-cell receptor-CD3 expression in enteropathy-associated T-cell lymphoma. Blood. 2008;112:5103–10.

40. Jabri B, De Serre NPM, Cellier C, et al. Selective expansion of intraepithelial lymphocytes expressing the HLA-E-specific natural killer receptor CD94 in celiac disease. Gastroenterology. 2000;118:867–79.

41. Mikulak J, Oriolo F, Bruni E, et al. NKp46-expressing human gut-resident intraepithelial Vδ1 T cell subpopulation exhibits high antitumor activity against colorectal cancer. JCI Insight. 2019;4:e125884.

42. Mayassi T, Ladell K, Gudjonson H, et al. Chronic inflammation permanently reshapes tissue-resident immunity in celiac disease. Cell. 2019;176:967–81.e19.

43. Cheminant M, Bruneau J, Malamut G, et al. NKp46 is a diagnostic biomarker and may be a therapeutic target in gastrointestinal T-cell lymphoproliferative diseases: a CELAC study. Gut. 2019;68:1396–405.

44. Tjon JM-L, Kooy-Winkelaar YMC, Tack GJ, et al. DNAM-1 mediates epithelial cell-specific cytotoxicity of aberrant intraepithelial lymphocyte lines from refractory celiac disease type II patients. J Immunol. 2011;186:6304–12.

45. Jabri B, Meresse B, Lee L, et al. Activating CD94 receptors which reduce the activation threshold of intraepithelial lymphocytes (IEL) are upregulated in celiac disease. Gastroenterology. 2002;122:A15–6.

46. Jarry A, Cerf-Bensussan N, Brousse N, et al. Subsets of CD3+ (T cell receptor alpha/beta or gamma/delta) and CD3- lymphocytes isolated from normal human gut epithelium display phenotypical features different from their counterparts in peripheral blood. Eur J Immunol. 1990;20:1097–103.

47. De Smedt M, Taghon T, Van de Walle I, et al. Notch signaling induces cytoplasmic CD3 epsilon expression in human differentiating NK cells. Blood. 2007;110:2696–703.

48. Guy-Grand D, Azogui O, Celli S, et al. Extrathymic T cell lymphopoiesis: ontogeny and contribution to gut intraepithelial lymphocytes in athymic and euthymic mice. J Exp Med. 2003;197:333–41.

49. Lambolez F, Azogui O, Joret A-M, et al. Characterization of T cell differentiation in the murine gut. J Exp Med. 2002;195:437–49.

50. Lin T, Matsuzaki G, Kenai H, et al. Progenies of fetal thymocytes are the major source of CD4-CD8+ alpha alpha intestinal intraepithelial lymphocytes early in ontogeny. Eur J Immunol. 1994;24:1785–91.

51. Shimizu H, Okamoto R, Ito G, et al. Distinct expression patterns of notch ligands, Dll1 and Dll4, in normal and inflamed mice intestine. PeerJ. 2014;2:e370.

52. van Wanrooij RLJ, de Jong D, Langerak AW, et al. Novel variant of EATL evolving from mucosal γδ-T-cells in a patient with type I RCD. BMJ Open Gastroenterol. 2015;2:e000026.

53. Malamut G, El Machhour R, Montcuquet N, et al. IL-15 triggers an antiapoptotic pathway in human intraepithelial lymphocytes that is a potential new target in celiac disease–associated inflammation and lymphomagenesis. J Clin Invest. 2010;120:2131–43.

54. Lio C-WJ, Yuita H, Rao A. Dysregulation of the TET family of epigenetic regulators in lymphoid and myeloid malignancies. Blood. 2019;134:1487–97.

55. Rao RC, Dou Y. Hijacked in cancer: the KMT2 (MLL) family of methyltransferases. Nat Rev Cancer. 2015;15:334–46.

56. Bol GM, Xie M, Raman V. DDX3, a potential target for cancer treatment. Mol Cancer. 2015;14:188.

57. Vogel TP, Milner JD, Cooper MA. The Ying and Yang of STAT3 in human disease. J Clin Immunol. 2015;35:615–23.

58. Hillmer EJ, Zhang H, Li HS, et al. STAT3 signaling in immunity introduction: STAT3 discovery, structure and transcriptional function. Cytokine Growth Factor Rev. 2016;31:1–15.

59. de Araujo ED, Orlova A, Neubauer HA, et al. Structural implications of STAT3 and STAT5 SH2 domain mutations. Cancers (Basel). 2019;11:1757.

60. Lamy T, Moignet A, Loughran TP. LGL leukemia: from pathogenesis to treatment. Blood. 2017;129:1082–94.

61. Liau NPD, Laktyushin A, Lucet IS, et al. The molecular basis of JAK/STAT inhibition by SOCS1. Nat Commun. 2018;9:1558.
62. Nilsen EM, Jahnsen FL, Lundin KE, et al. Gluten induces an intestinal cytokine response strongly dominated by interferon gamma in patients with celiac disease. Gastroenterology. 1998;115:551–63.
63. Bodd M, Raki M, Tollefsen S, et al. HLA-DQ2-restricted gluten-reactive T cells produce IL-21 but not IL-17 or IL-22. Mucosal Immunol. 2010;3:594–601.
64. Verstrepen L, Carpentier I, Verhelst K, et al. ABINs: A20 binding inhibitors of NF-κB and apoptosis signaling. Biochem Pharmacol. 2009;78:105–14.
65. Hymowitz SG, Wertz IE. A20: from ubiquitin editing to tumour suppression. Nat Rev Cancer. 2010;10:332–40.
66. Charbit-Henrion F, Parlato M, Malamut G, et al. Intestinal immunoregulation: lessons from human mendelian diseases. Mucosal Immunol. 2021;14(5):1017–37.
67. Grivennikov SI, Karin M. Dangerous liaisons: STAT3 and NF-κB collaboration and crosstalk in cancer. Cytokine Growth Factor Rev. 2010;21:11–9.
68. Kooy-Winkelaar YMC, Bouwer D, Janssen GMC, et al. CD4 T-cell cytokines synergize to induce proliferation of malignant and nonmalignant innate intraepithelial lymphocytes. Proc Natl Acad Sci. 2017;114:E980–9.
69. O'Keeffe J, Lynch S, Whelan A, et al. Flow cytometric measurement of intracellular migration inhibition factor and tumour necrosis factor alpha in the mucosa of patients with coeliac disease. Clin Exp Immunol. 2001;125:376–82.
70. Baran-Marszak F, Boukhiar M, Harel S, et al. Constitutive and B-cell receptor-induced activation of STAT3 are important signaling pathways targeted by bortezomib in leukemic mantle cell lymphoma. Haematologica. 2010;95:1865–72.
71. Soderquist CR, Lewis SK, Gru AA, et al. Immunophenotypic spectrum and genomic landscape of refractory celiac disease type II. Am J Surg Pathol. 2021;45(7):905–16.
72. Crescenzo R, Abate F, Lasorsa E, et al. Convergent mutations and kinase fusions lead to oncogenic STAT3 activation in anaplastic large cell lymphoma. Cancer Cell. 2015;27:516–32.
73. Roberti A, Dobay MP, Bisig B, et al. Type II enteropathy-associated T-cell lymphoma features a unique genomic profile with highly recurrent SETD2 alterations. Nat Commun. 2016;7:12602.
74. Sharma A, Oishi N, Boddicker RL, et al. Recurrent STAT3-JAK2 fusions in indolent T-cell lymphoproliferative disorder of the gastrointestinal tract. Blood. 2018;131:2262–6.
75. Soderquist CR, Patel N, Murty VV, et al. Genetic and phenotypic characterization of indolent T-cell lymphoproliferative disorders of the gastrointestinal tract. Haematologica. 2019;105(7):1895–906.
76. Nairismägi M-L, Tan J, Lim JQ, et al. JAK-STAT and G-protein-coupled receptor signaling pathways are frequently altered in epitheliotropic intestinal T-cell lymphoma. Leukemia. 2016;30:1311–9.
77. Moffitt AB, Ondrejka SL, McKinney M, et al. Enteropathy-associated T cell lymphoma subtypes are characterized by loss of function of SETD2. J Exp Med. 2017;214:1371–86.
78. Laurent C, Nicolae A, Laurent C, et al. Gene alterations in epigenetic modifiers and JAK-STAT signaling are frequent in breast implant-associated ALCL. Blood. 2020;135(5):360–70.
79. Al–toma A, Goerres MS, JWR M, et al. Cladribine therapy in refractory celiac disease with aberrant T cells. Clin Gastroenterol Hepatol. 2006;4:1322–7.
80. Goodman GR, Beutler E, Saven A. Cladribine in the treatment of hairy-cell leukaemia. Best Pract Res Clin Haematol. 2003;16:101–16.
81. Nijeboer P, Wanrooij R, Gils T, et al. Lymphoma development and survival in refractory coeliac disease type II: histological response as prognostic factor. United Eur Gastroenterol J. 2017;5:208–17.
82. Vivas S, de Morales JMR, Ramos F, et al. Alemtuzumab for refractory celiac disease in a patient at risk for enteropathy-associated T-cell lymphoma. N Engl J Med. 2006;354:2514–5.

83. Cheminant M, Bruneau J, Malamut G, et al. NKp46 is a diagnostic biomarker and may be a therapeutic target in gastrointestinal T-cell lymphoproliferative diseases: A CELAC study. Gut. 2018;68:1396–405.
84. Mukewar SS, Sharma A, Rubio-Tapia A, et al. Open-capsule budesonide for refractory celiac disease. Am J Gastroenterol. 2017;112:959–67.
85. Cellier C, Bouma G, van Gils T, et al. Safety and efficacy of AMG 714 in patients with type 2 refractory coeliac disease: a phase 2a, randomised, double-blind, placebo-controlled, parallel-group study. Lancet Gastroenterol Hepatol. 2019;4:960–70.
86. Zhang S, Zhao J, Bai X, et al. Biological effects of IL-15 on immune cells and its potential for the treatment of cancer. Int Immunopharmacol. 2021;91:107318.
87. Song TL, Nairismägi M-L, Laurensia Y, et al. Oncogenic activation of the STAT3 pathway drives PD-L1 expression in natural killer/T-cell lymphoma. Blood. 2018;132:1146–58.
88. Kivelä L, Caminero A, Leffler DA, et al. Current and emerging therapies for coeliac disease. Nat Rev Gastroenterol Hepatol. 2021;18:181–95.
89. Tack GJ, Wondergem MJ, Al-Toma A, et al. Auto-SCT in refractory celiac disease type II patients unresponsive to cladribine therapy. Bone Marrow Transplant. 2011;46:840–6.
90. Du M-Q. MALT lymphoma: genetic abnormalities, immunological stimulation and molecular mechanism. Best Pract Res Clin Haematol. 2017;30:13–23.
91. Malamut G, Meresse B, Kaltenbach S, et al. Small intestinal CD4+ T-cell lymphoma is a heterogenous entity with common pathology features. Clin Gastroenterol Hepatol. 2014;12:599–608.e1.

# From Unresponsive Celiac Disease to Refractory Celiac Disease: Epidemiological Data

Knut E. A. Lundin and Katri Kaukinen

## Introduction

The outcome(s) of dietary treatment of celiac disease (CD) is in most patients usually good in terms of clinical response measured by Patient Reported Outcome Measures (PROMs), healing of the mucosa and healing of the associated osteoporosis among may other aspects of the disease. Unfortunately, not all patients experience this improvement. In some cases, the patient experience first a beneficial response, then to deteriorate. Lack of response may be due to poor compliance either because the patient lack knowledge on the gluten free diet or motivation to follow the diet, and it is of utmost importance to sort this question out.

Most experts would agree that a strict gluten-free diet for at least six months is needed before so-called refractory CD (RCD) can be considered [1–3]. However, even this time frame is too short for full mucosal healing as this in most adults require longer time (Table 1) [4, 5]. This, together with a clear definition (so called "gold standard") of RCD hampers precise studies on the epidemiology of the disorder. It can further bluntly be stated that too many clinicians diagnose RCD when the matter is only that there is slow and incomplete mucosal healing in a relatively well-doing patient.

The distinction of RCD into two types, 1 and 2, was proposed based on seminal work particularly by the research groups of Christophe Cellier in Paris and Chris

K. E. A. Lundin (✉)
Stiftelsen KG Jebsen Coeliac Disease Research Centre, Faculty of Medicine, University of Oslo, Oslo, Norway

Department of Gastroenterology, Oslo University Hospital Rikshospitalet, Oslo, Norway
e-mail: knut.lundin@medisin.uio.no

K. Kaukinen
Faculty of Medicine and Health Technology, Tampere University and Department of Internal Medicine Tampere University Hospital, Tampere, Finland
e-mail: katri.kaukinen@tuni.fi

© Springer Nature Switzerland AG 2022
G. Malamut, N. Cerf-Bensussan (eds.), *Refractory Celiac Disease*,
https://doi.org/10.1007/978-3-030-90142-4_4

**Table 1** Studies on small bowel mucosal histological recovery rates (%) and proportion of celiac disease (CD) patients with persistent villous atrophy on a gluten-free diet (GFD)

| Ref. | Year | Country | CD, n | Duration of GFD, years (median) | Mucosal recovery/ improvement | Persistent villous atrophy |
|---|---|---|---|---|---|---|
| [19] | 2003 | USA | 39 | 8.5[a] | 21% | 79% |
| [20] | 2007 | Italy | 114 | 2 | 38% | 62% |
| [21] | 2021 | Spain | 76 | 2 | 47% | 53% |
| [5] | 2016 | Norway | 127 | 1.1 | 51% | 49% |
| [23] | 2010 | UK | 284 | 1.6 | 56% | 44% |
| [48] | 2014 | Sweden | 7648 | 1.3 | 57% | 43% |
| [4] | 2002 | Netherlands | 158 | <2 | 65% | 35% |
| [25] | 2015 | Finland | 263 | 1 | 68% | 32% |
| [11] | 2002 | Italy | 390 | 6.9[a] | 76% | 24% |
| [27] | 2009 | Italy | 465 | 1.3[a] | 79% | 21% |
| [28] | 2016 | Australia | 46 | 5 | 85% | 15% |
| [29] | 2010 | USA | 241 | <2 | 88% | 12% |
| [4] | 2002 | Netherlands | 158 | >5 | 90% | 10% |
| [5] | 2016 | Norway | 127 | 8.1 | 94% | 6% |
| [30] | 2012 | Finland | 177 | 11[a] | 96% | 4% |

[a]Mean

Mulder in Amsterdam [6, 7]. The type 2 is by definition a condition with one (or some very few) dominant monoclonal T cell population—and unfortunately frequent transition to an overt Enteropathy Associated T cell Lymphoma (EATL) with dismal prognosis. Such a situation was known before the turn of the century bases on work by Isaacson and others [8, 9]. At first glance, it seems "easy" to diagnose RCD type 2, but as detailed elsewhere in this book, that is certainly not the case. The type 1 RCD is even more difficult to define. In this chapter, we will discuss the Type 1 and Type 2 mostly separately.

# The Problems with Investigating Compliance

For the un-involved, it might seem easy to attend a gluten-free diet and indeed many CD patients cope with this with success. However, it has repeatedly been shown that many patients struggle and poor compliance is a major problem [10, 11]. The in-depth interview by a trained clinical dietician has to this end been the main method for checking compliance. Structured scoring forms have been developed and is of great help [12–14].

More recently, an attempt to develop an objective tool has been developed addressing gluten peptides in urine and feces [15]. It turns out that gluten peptides can be detected in urine for some hours after intake of regular food, and in feces for some days. It is obvious that the urine test has some advantages for practical reasons. The main message from clinical testing of these assays is that gluten exposure is more frequent than previously considered and that it correlates with mucosal damage [16, 17]. However, also conflicting results have been reported and not all investigators embrace this new method [18].

## Mucosal Healing and Outcome

While elimination of gluten from the diet improves the villous architecture and reduces the number of intraepithelial lymphocytes in celiac disease, several studies show an incomplete histological normalization of small intestinal mucosa despite patients adhering to a strict gluten-free diet (Table 1) [4, 5, 19–30]. This might suggest inadvertent gluten intake, but it is also known that in approximately half of the adult patients it takes more than 1–2 years before mucosal recovery is achieved. More severe disease in terms of histology and serology and signs of malabsorption at diagnosis have predicted delayed mucosal healing [25]. Interestingly, incomplete villous recovery and the speed of mucosal healing in repeat biopsy after 1 year on a gluten-free diet seems not to affect the short- or long-term clinical outcomes [5, 25]. However, persistent villous atrophy has been associated with a risk of complications such as fractures [31] and the development of lymphomas [32] suggesting that mucosal healing could be an endpoint in assessment of the response to the gluten-free diet. Although a repeat biopsy during a gluten-free diet is currently the only reliable tool to demonstrate mucosal healing, there are no studies indicating an absolute necessity for performing routine follow-up biopsy for all celiac disease patients. Owing to this ambiguity, in the current ESSCD [3] and BSG [2] guidelines there is no consensus on the recommendation of routine use of biopsy in adults.

## Epidemiology of RCD1

In rare cases persistent small bowel mucosal villous atrophy on a strict gluten-free diet indicates refractory celiac disease. The literature on the epidemiology of refractory celiac disease is scarce and often limited to a few studies from tertiary referral centers (Table 2) [4, 22, 33–40]. Recent population representative studies indicate that the prevalence of refractory celiac disease is only 0.3–0.5% among celiac disease patients [35, 38–40] and 0.002% in the general population [40]. Patients of male gender, older age, severe symptoms or seronegativity at the diagnosis of celiac disease as well as those having previous history of dietary transgressions are at risk of future refractory celiac disease [40]. RCD1 is more commonly diagnosed in the US, whereas the first European-published series of RCD patients reported high

**Table 2** Studies on the prevalence of refractory celiac disease (RCD) among CD patients

| Ref. | Year | Country | Celiac disease, n | RCD, n | Prevalence of RCD | Proportion of RCD2 cases out of all RCD patients |
|------|------|---------|-------------------|--------|-------------------|--------------------------------------------------|
| [33] | 2013 | USA | 700 | 73 | 10% | 9% |
| [4] | 2002 | Netherlands | 158 | 11 | 7% | ND |
| [34] | 2010 | USA | 844 | 34 | 4% | 15% |
| [35] | 2017 | Austria | 1138 | 29 | 3.3%−>0.5% | 24% |
| [36] | 2007 | USA | 603 | 10 | 1.7% | ND |
| [22] | 2010 | USA | 204 | 3 | 1.5% | 33% |
| [37] | 2009 | UK | 713 | 5 | 0.7% | 100% |
| [38] | 2013 | UK | 391 | 2 | 0.4% | 0% |
| [39] | 2014 | Italy | 1835 | 9 | 0.5% | 22% |
| [40] | 2014 | Finland | 12,240 | 38 | 0.3% | 23% |

*ND*, not defined

percentages of RCD2 patients (28–75%) among all RCD patients [41–43]. However, recent population based studies suggest that RCD1 predominates also in Europe (Table 2).

# Epidemiology of RCD2

Since its first descriptions, RCD2 has intrigued scientists and attracted considerable attention in the CD research field [44]. This is not the least because of the dismal prognosis of the disorder with 5-year survival rates around 50% [22, 45, 46]. However, almost all cases of RCD2 have been carefully collected in regional or national competence and tertiary referral centres so the population prevalence figures are rather uncertain. At any rate, the disorder is not at all frequent. The case of Holland illustrates this, where Chris Mulder and colleagues for years have actively collected new cases by repeated questionnaires to fellow gastroenterologists [47]. During a 6-year period from 2006 and 2012, not more than 13 cases of RCD2 were collected in addition to 20 patients with RCD1, yielding an annual incidence of 0.83/10,000 CeD patients. Similar findings were done in Finland using the same methodology involving 11 hospital districts [40]. Out of 44 patients that received the RCD diagnosis, 68% had RCD1 and 23% had RCD2, in 9% of the cases the type could not be determined. This is a country with a very high detection rate for CeD. They concluded that the prevalence of RCD was 0.31% among diagnosed CeD patients and 0.002% in the general population. It is interesting to note that RCD2 is never seen in children and with extremely few exceptions not seen in adults below the age of 50–60. This suggests that duration of untreated disease may play an important role in the pathogenesis, given that the RCD2 patients may have gone with undetected disease. However, occurrence of RCD2 also in patients with well treated CD for years may happen.

## Concluding Remarks

Refractory celiac disease is a serious but fortunately rather rare condition. Slow and incomplete mucosal healing in "regular" CD" is often confused with RCD. RCD type 1 lacks clear definitions, whereas diagnosis of RCD type 2 relies on mucosal immunopathology and molecular biology investigations. The rarity of the condition and lack of effective treatment options calls for centralized care.

## References

1. Ryan BM, Kelleher D. Refractory celiac disease. Gastroenterology. 2000;119(1):243–51.
2. Ludvigsson JF, et al. Diagnosis and management of adult coeliac disease: guidelines from the British Society of Gastroenterology. Gut. 2014;63(8):1210–28.
3. Al-Toma A, et al. European Society for the Study of Coeliac Disease (ESsCD) guideline for coeliac disease and other gluten-related disorders. United European Gastroenterol J. 2019;7(5):583–613.
4. Wahab PJ, Meijer JW, Mulder CJ. Histologic follow-up of people with celiac disease on a gluten-free diet: slow and incomplete recovery. Am J Clin Pathol. 2002;118(3):459–63.
5. Haere P, et al. Long-term mucosal recovery and healing in celiac disease is the rule - not the exception. Scand J Gastroenterol. 2016;51(12):1439–46.
6. Cellier C, et al. Refractory sprue, coeliac disease, and enteropathy-associated T-cell lymphoma. French Coeliac Disease Study Group. Lancet. 2000;356(9225):203–8.
7. Mulder CJ, et al. Refractory coeliac disease: a window between coeliac disease and enteropathy associated T cell lymphoma. Scand J Gastroenterol Suppl. 2000;232:32–7.
8. Isaacson PG, et al. Malignant histiocytosis of the intestine: a T-cell lymphoma. Lancet. 1985;2(8457):688–91.
9. Alfsen GC, et al. Low-grade intestinal lymphoma of intraepithelial T lymphocytes with concomitant enteropathy-associated T cell lymphoma: case report suggesting a possible histogenetic relationship. Hum Pathol. 1989;20(9):909–13.
10. Freeman HJ. Dietary compliance in celiac disease. World J Gastroenterol. 2017;23(15):2635–9.
11. Silvester JA, et al. Most patients with celiac disease on gluten-free diets consume measurable amounts of gluten. Gastroenterology. 2020;158(5):1497–99.e1.
12. Leffler DA, et al. A simple validated gluten-free diet adherence survey for adults with celiac disease. Clin Gastroenterol Hepatol. 2009;7(5):530–6. 536.e1–2
13. Gladys K, et al. Celiac dietary adherence test and standardized dietician evaluation in assessment of adherence to a gluten-free diet in patients with celiac disease. Nutrients. 2020;12(8):2300.
14. Biagi F, et al. A gluten-free diet score to evaluate dietary compliance in patients with coeliac disease. Br J Nutr. 2009;102(6):882–7.
15. Comino I, et al. Fecal gluten peptides reveal limitations of serological tests and food questionnaires for monitoring gluten-free diet in celiac disease patients. Am J Gastroenterol. 2016;111(10):1456–65.
16. Moreno ML, et al. Detection of gluten immunogenic peptides in the urine of patients with coeliac disease reveals transgressions in the gluten-free diet and incomplete mucosal healing. Gut. 2017;66(2):250–7.
17. Ruiz-Carnicer A, et al. Negative predictive value of the repeated absence of gluten immunogenic peptides in the urine of treated celiac patients in predicting mucosal healing: new proposals for follow-up in celiac disease. Am J Clin Nutr. 2020;112(5):1240–51.

18. Laserna-Mendieta EJ, et al. Poor sensitivity of fecal gluten immunogenic peptides and serum antibodies to detect duodenal mucosal damage in celiac disease monitoring. Nutrients. 2020;13(1):98.
19. Lee SK, et al. Duodenal histology in patients with celiac disease after treatment with a gluten-free diet. Gastrointest Endosc. 2003;57(2):187–91.
20. Bardella MT, et al. Coeliac disease: a histological follow-up study. Histopathology. 2007;50(4):465–71.
21. Fernandez-Banares F, et al. Persistent villous atrophy in de novo adult patients with celiac disease and strict control of gluten-free diet adherence: a multicenter prospective study (CADER study). Am J Gastroenterol. 2021;116(5):1036–43.
22. Rubio-Tapia A, Murray JA. Classification and management of refractory coeliac disease. Gut. 2010;59(4):547–57.
23. Hutchinson JM, et al. Long-term histological follow-up of people with coeliac disease in a UK teaching hospital. QJM. 2010;103(7):511–7.
24. Lebwohl B, et al. Predictors of persistent villous atrophy in coeliac disease: a population-based study. Aliment Pharmacol Ther. 2014;39(5):488–95.
25. Pekki H, et al. Predictors and significance of incomplete mucosal recovery in celiac disease after 1 year on a gluten-free diet. Am J Gastroenterol. 2015;110(7):1078–85.
26. Ciacci C, et al. Long-term follow-up of celiac adults on gluten-free diet: prevalence and correlates of intestinal damage. Digestion. 2002;66(3):178–85.
27. Lanzini A, et al. Complete recovery of intestinal mucosa occurs very rarely in adult coeliac patients despite adherence to gluten-free diet. Aliment Pharmacol Ther. 2009;29(12):1299–308.
28. Newnham ED, et al. Adherence to the gluten-free diet can achieve the therapeutic goals in almost all patients with coeliac disease: a 5-year longitudinal study from diagnosis. J Gastroenterol Hepatol. 2016;31(2):342–9.
29. Rubio-Tapia A, et al. Mucosal recovery and mortality in adults with celiac disease after treatment with a gluten-free diet. Am J Gastroenterol. 2010;105(6):1412–20.
30. Tuire I, et al. Persistent duodenal intraepithelial lymphocytosis despite a long-term strict gluten-free diet in celiac disease. Am J Gastroenterol. 2012;107(10):1563–9.
31. Lebwohl B, et al. Persistent mucosal damage and risk of fracture in celiac disease. J Clin Endocrinol Metab. 2014;99(2):609–16.
32. Lebwohl B, et al. Mucosal healing and risk for lymphoproliferative malignancy in celiac disease: a population-based cohort study. Ann Intern Med. 2013;159(3):169–75.
33. Arguelles-Grande C, et al. Immunohistochemical and T-cell receptor gene rearrangement analyses as predictors of morbidity and mortality in refractory celiac disease. J Clin Gastroenterol. 2013;47(7):593–601.
34. Roshan B, et al. The incidence and clinical spectrum of refractory celiac disease in a north american referral center. Am J Gastroenterol. 2011;106(5):923–8.
35. Eigner W, et al. Dynamics of occurrence of refractory coeliac disease and associated complications over 25 years. Aliment Pharmacol Ther. 2017;45(2):364–72.
36. Leffler DA, et al. Etiologies and predictors of diagnosis in nonresponsive celiac disease. Clin Gastroenterol Hepatol. 2007;5(4):445–50.
37. West J. Celiac disease and its complications: a time traveller's perspective. Gastroenterology. 2009;136(1):32–4.
38. Sharkey LM, et al. Optimising delivery of care in coeliac disease - comparison of the benefits of repeat biopsy and serological follow-up. Aliment Pharmacol Ther. 2013;38(10):1278–91.
39. Biagi F, et al. Low incidence but poor prognosis of complicated coeliac disease: a retrospective multicentre study. Dig Liver Dis. 2014;46(3):227–30.
40. Ilus T, et al. Refractory coeliac disease in a country with a high prevalence of clinically-diagnosed coeliac disease. Aliment Pharmacol Ther. 2014;39(4):418–25.
41. Al-Toma A, et al. Survival in refractory coeliac disease and enteropathy-associated T-cell lymphoma: retrospective evaluation of single-centre experience. Gut. 2007;56(10):1373–8.

42. Daum S, et al. High rates of complications and substantial mortality in both types of refractory sprue. Eur J Gastroenterol Hepatol. 2009;21(1):66–70.
43. Malamut G, et al. Presentation and long-term follow-up of refractory celiac disease: comparison of type I with type II. Gastroenterology. 2009;136(1):81–90.
44. Baggus EMR, et al. How to manage adult coeliac disease: perspective from the NHS England Rare Diseases Collaborative Network for Non-Responsive and Refractory Coeliac Disease. Frontline Gastroenterol. 2020;11(3):235–42.
45. Malamut G, Cellier C. Refractory celiac disease. Expert Rev Gastroenterol Hepatol. 2014;8(3):323–8.
46. Rubio-Tapia A, et al. Creation of a model to predict survival in patients with refractory coeliac disease using a multinational registry. Aliment Pharmacol Ther. 2016;44(7):704–14.
47. van Wanrooij RL, et al. Outcome of referrals for non-responsive celiac disease in a tertiary center: low incidence of refractory celiac disease in the Netherlands. Clin Transl Gastroenterol. 2017;8(1):e218.
48. Al-Toma A, Verbeek WH, Mulder CJ. Update on the management of refractory coeliac disease. J Gastrointestin Liver Dis. 2007;16(1):57–63.

# The Role of Endoscopy in Refractory Coeliac Disease

H. A. Penny, S. Chetcuti Zammat, R. Sidhu, and D. S. Sanders

## Introduction

Per-oral small bowel (SB) biopsy has been the foundation in the diagnosis of coeliac disease (CD) since the development of the Crosby capsule in the 1960s [1]. Since then, technological advances have enabled refinement of endoscopic practice and image [2]. The application of oesophagogastroduodenoscopy, or upper gastrointestinal (GI) endoscopy, allows for real-time visualisation of mucosal irregularities and obtaining targeted small bowel (SB) biopsies [2]. The recent development of small bowel capsule endoscopy (SBCE) has enabled inspection of the SB beyond the reach of a standard gastroscope, with minimal inconvenience to patients [3]. Mucosal irregularities detected by SBCE distal to the duodenum can subsequently be biopsied using more invasive enteroscopic techniques, such as device-assisted enteroscopy (DAE).

In uncomplicated CD, upper GI endoscopy with duodenal biopsies remains the gold standard endoscopic approach for diagnosis [4]. Studies support the use of SBCE in individuals who have raised anti-endomysial and/or anti-tissue transglutaminase antibody titres who are unwilling, or unable to undergo upper GI endoscopy [5]. Additionally, the mucosal irregularities in CD can be patchy and isolated to the mid or distal SB, hence SBCE and enteroscopy can be employed in cases of diagnostic uncertainty in uncomplicated CD, or when there is discordance between clinical suspicion and duodenal histology [6, 7].

H. A. Penny (✉) · S. Chetcuti Zammat · R. Sidhu · D. S. Sanders
Academic Unit of Gastroenterology, University of Sheffield, Sheffield, UK
e-mail: h.penny@sheffield.ac.uk; reenasidhu@nhs.net; David.Sanders@sth.nhs.uk

© Springer Nature Switzerland AG 2022
G. Malamut, N. Cerf-Bensussan (eds.), *Refractory Celiac Disease*,
https://doi.org/10.1007/978-3-030-90142-4_5

Approximately 0.3–10% of individuals with CD will develop refractory CD (RCD) [8–10], which is defined as the presence of ongoing SB mucosal inflammation typical of CD despite strict removal of gluten from the diet for at least 12 months [11].There are two types of RCD: RCD I and RCD II. The two subtypes are differentiated based on the presence of an abnormal expansion of an "aberrant" subset of small intestinal intraepithelial lymphocytes (IELs), which is detected in RCD II [9]. Individuals with RCD, particularly RCD II, have an increased risk of developing complications such as ulcerative jejunitis and enteropathy associated T cell lymphoma (EATL) [8–10]. As such, 5-year survival in RCD II is around 50%, compared with 90%–100% in patients with RCD I [3, 8–10]. Mucosal inflammation associated with RCD and associated pre-malignant/malignant lesions can affect anywhere along the length of the small intestine [9, 10]. Therefore, endoscopic evaluation of the entire length of the SB is essential when assessing individuals with suspicion for RCD [12]. It is also important to assess the length of the SB in those with established RCD at regular intervals, to monitor for the development of pre-malignant/malignant lesions [12]. This chapter provides an overview of the literature surrounding the use of SB endoscopy in RCD.

## Upper GI Endoscopy

RCD is diagnosed on the presence of persisting or recurring SB villous atrophy, intra-epithelial lymphocytosis and crypt hyperplasia (Marsh III lesions) despite strict adherence to a gluten-free diet (GFD) [11]. Thus, an important step in the assessment of individuals with suspected RCD is to determine whether histological changes typical of CD persist. Upper GI endoscopy with up-to-date duodenal biopsies is an appropriate initial approach, owing to widespread availability of this test. However, distinguishing whether persisting changes are due to ongoing gluten exposure, slow mucosal healing, or RCD I on duodenal biopsies alone is difficult and requires careful assessment of clinical presentation and dietary history [12]. Other causes of villous atrophy[1] should also be considered in individuals before attributing these findings to persistent CD. In contrast, RCD II can be identified by determining the characteristic expansion of aberrant IELs on duodenal biopsies, using flow cytometry or immunohistochemistry [13].

Numerous studies have highlighted the importance of the site, method, number and orientation of duodenal biopsies sampled during upper GI endoscopy to enable an accurate diagnosis of uncomplicated CD [7, 14–16]. To this end, guidelines recommend that a minimum of four single-bite biopsies are taken from the duodenum with at least one from the duodenal bulb [4]. The importance of biopsy acquisition, handling and assessment has not been assessed specifically in the

---

[1] Other causes of villous atrophy include immune-mediated (e.g. autoimmune enteropathy), immune deficiency (e.g. CVID), inflammatory (e.g. eosinophilic gastroenteritis, IBD), infectious (e.g. giardiasis), iatrogenic (e.g. NSAIDs) and idiopathic [4].

setting of RCD. However, it seems appropriate that the same standards of duodenal biopsy sampling are applied in the setting of suspected RCD, as in uncomplicated CD, to enable accurate assessment of mucosal inflammation in these individuals.

## Small Bowel Capsule Endoscopy

The inflammation in RCD can be patchy and the associated pre-malignant/malignant lesions are primarily located in the jejunum but may also affect the distal SB [17–19]. Therefore, endoscopic inspection of the entire length of the SB, by oesophago-gastro-duodenoscopy (OGD) and SBCE, is essential in suspected RCD (Fig. 1).

SBCE is a minimally invasive endoscopic method which produces high quality images of the SB with an eight-fold magnification [20]. The high magnification and clarity of the images enables accurate assessment of the SB mucosa and detection

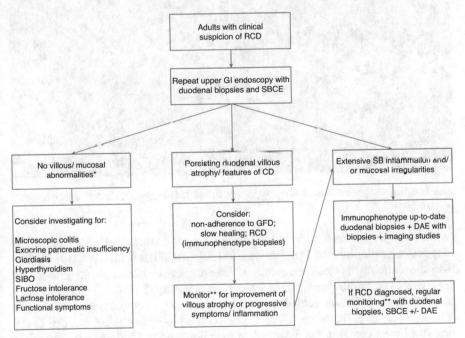

**Fig. 1** Flow chart outlining the endoscopic assessment of adults with clinical suspicion for RCD. *Patients with CD can present with apparent non-responsiveness, but their symptoms can rather be the result of conditions associated with CD [12]. Therefore, where no villous/mucosal abnormalities are detected, other conditions associated with CD should be considered in individuals with persisting symptoms. **Currently, there is no consensus on the interval for monitoring individuals considered to have persisting villous atrophy secondary to ongoing gluten exposure or slow healing. UK experts recommend a 12-monthly monitoring interval for patients with RCD I once treatment response is established and a 6-monthly interval for patients with RCD II

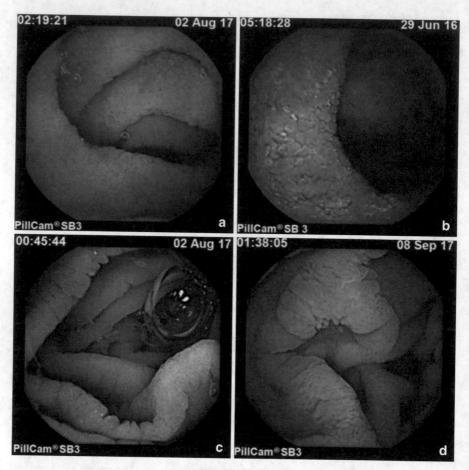

**Fig. 2** SBCE images consistent with (**a**), villous atrophy; (**b**), mosaicism; (**c**), scalloping; (**d**), fissuring

of macroscopic villous atrophy as well as endoscopic features typical of CD such as mosaicism, scalloping and fissuring (Fig. 2) [20]. SBCE has been shown to be better than conventional upper GI endoscopy at detecting these endoscopic features of CD [21]. However, studies have reported variable sensitivity (70–100%) and specificity (64–100%) of SBCE for achieving a diagnosis of CD, in comparison to duodenal histology [22–25]. Therefore, SBCE is not routinely used in clinical practice as the first-line investigation in the diagnosis of uncomplicated CD. Rather, it is reserved for those who are unwilling or unable to undergo upper GI endoscopy, or individuals with a high index of suspicion for CD, who have normal duodenal biopsies [26].

In contrast, SBCE is recommended in individuals with suspected or established RCD to evaluate the presence of SB mucosal irregularities associated with

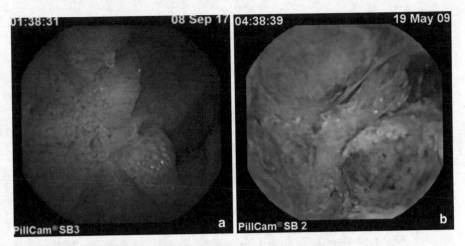

**Fig. 3** SBCE images consistent with (**a**), mucosal ulcerations; (**b**), EATL

pre-malignant/malignant complications (Fig. 3) [25]. In a recent multicentre study of 189 patients with established coeliac disease who had new or persisting symptoms, SBCE had a diagnostic yield of 67.2% for mucosal abnormalities including villous atrophy, ulcers and lymphoma. Notably, the findings from SBCE modified management in 59.3% of the cases [27]. Other studies, in patients with established CD and persisting symptoms, have also reported the usefulness of SBCE in detecting macroscopic villous atrophy, ulcerative jejunoileitis, lymphoma and adeno-carcinoma in these patients [21, 28, 29]. Importantly, in a number of cases, these lesions were undetectable by upper GI endoscopy [27]. Thus, a dual endoscopic approach (i.e. OGD and SBCE) is essential in the assessment of suspected or established RCD.

Studies using SBCE have also reported that individuals with RCD have a greater percentage and longer length of small intestinal mucosal inflammation than individuals with uncomplicated CD [21, 30]. Patients with RCD were also shown to have significantly more scalloping of the mucosa and SB ulcers than those with uncomplicated CD [30]. In addition, those with RCD II were found to have more extensive lesions involving the distal jejunum and ileum on SBCE than patients with RCD I [21]. Therefore, the demonstration of extensive SB inflammation on SBCE may help identify individuals with RCD.

Moreover, evaluating disease extent by SBCE may provide information about response to treatment in RCD. In this manner, comparing the extent and length of SB inflammation on consecutive tests, may inform on mucosal healing, or persistent/worsening disease [20]. Indeed, a recent study reported that the percentage of SB mucosa affected in patients with RCD decreased in 61% (14/23) of patients, from an average of 42.4% to 26.4%, following treatment [30]. Intriguingly, there were no clear changes in the Marsh grade of duodenal biopsies in 87% (20/23) of cases at follow-up [30]. Therefore, reliance on histology alone to monitor for treatment response may be inaccurate. However, the clinical relevance of evaluating the extent of SB inflammation in uncomplicated CD is unclear [31, 32] and current guidelines do not recommend using SBCE to monitor response to a GFD in uncomplicated CD [26]. Therefore, further studies are awaited to assess the clinical usefulness of this approach in RCD.

Notably, there are limitations to SBCE, including the inability to take biopsies and that the interpretation of images is subjective, meaning that subtle villous abnormalities may not be identified [20]. Machine learning algorithms are being developed to aide with the interpretation of SBCE recordings and new generation capsule technology have improved optics to enhance the clarity and resolution of the capsule images [20]. Furthermore, one of the risks associated with this procedure is capsule retention within the intestines. Patients with RCD II, ulcerative lesions and EATL can have a significant risk of small-bowel structuring [33]. Patients should therefore undergo a prior patency capsule to reduce the incidence of capsule retention.

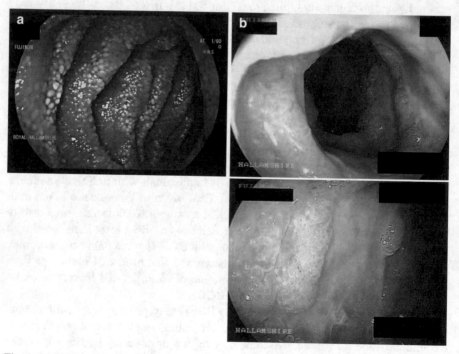

**Fig. 4** (a) DBE images from the mid-jejunum of an individual with SB lymphoma. (b) Top and bottom; DBE images of a patient with RCD II and raised mucosal patches

## Device Assisted Enteroscopy

Where SBCE has identified mucosal irregularities, more invasive enteroscopic techniques can be employed to obtain biopsy samples for histological assessment of lesions that are identified beyond the reach of a standard gastroscope (Fig. 4). Of the different enteroscopy approaches, DAE is preferred over push enteroscopy as it enables a greater depth of SB visualisation [26, 34]. DAE includes several techniques including double balloon enteroscopy (DBE), single balloon enteroscopy, spiral enteroscopy and balloon-guided endoscopy. The diagnostic yield and safety profile across different DAE techniques is similar [26]; although, within the RCD literature, DBE is most frequently used.

Three studies have illustrated the value of enteroscopy in RCD (Table 1). Most individuals across all three studies were enrolled in enteroscopy for histologic definition of lesions identified on SBCE [19, 35, 36]. Pooled analysis of these studies identified that around a third (27.7%) of the irregularities detected on SBCE represent pre-malignant/malignant lesions [37]. Therefore, while the use of DAE to define lesions identified by SBCE in patients with RCD is warranted [26], further characterisation of mucosal irregularities on SBCE which correlate with pre-malignant/ malignant lesions may help to improve patient selection for DAE. Other causes for SB ulcerative lesions include Crohn's disease, infections, or medication usage (including non-steroidal anti-inflammatory drugs) and these should be considered in the appropriate clinical context [20].

## Which Patients Should Undergo Endoscopy?

Patients with RCD often initially present to gastroenterology services with non-responsive CD—a broad term which refers to patients with persistent or relapsing symptoms typical of CD despite adherence to a GFD—although some individuals may be diagnosed with RCD II at the time of index CD diagnosis [12]. Non-responsiveness occurs in up to a third of individuals with CD and is most commonly

**Table 1** Studies evaluating enteroscopy in complicated and refractory CD (adapted from Ref. 37)

| Study | Total number of patients | Number of patients with RCD | Type of enteroscopy | Number of pre-malignant SB lesions detected | Number of malignant SB lesions detected |
|---|---|---|---|---|---|
| Cellier; 1999 [35] | 31 | 8 | Push enteroscopy | Five ulcerative jejunitis | 0 |
| Hadithi; 2007 [36] | 21 | 21 | DBE | Two ulcerative jejunitis | Five EATL |
| Tomba; 2016 [19] | 24 | 9 | DBE | Six ulcerative jejunitis | Two SB adenocarcinoma; one neuroendocrine tumour |

caused by continued gluten exposure (35–50% of cases) [38, 39], but may also be caused by slow mucosal healing, or gluten supersensitivity, or an alternative condition to CD [40]. By contrast, RCD collectively represents a minority of those with non-responsiveness (up to a quarter of patients investigated at specialist centres [9, 41–43], although the true prevalence is likely to be much lower [12, 38]), but is associated with more significant morbidity and mortality, which may be improved by prompt diagnosis [12]. All patients presenting with non-responsiveness should undergo a repeat OGD [40], however identifying those who should undergo full length endoscopic evaluation of the SB (i.e. OGD and SBCE) to evaluate for suspected RCD is less clear.

The literature suggests that those with RCD II and EATL are older (>50 years) individuals diagnosed with CD later in life [8, 42, 44]. A recent study found that 6/7 (85.7%) patients diagnosed with EATL presented with new "alarm" symptoms[2] [27]. Furthermore, a multicentre case-controlled study of 87 patients with complicated CD showed that EATL and ulcerative jejunitis were more frequent among individuals who had no remittance of their symptoms after index CD diagnosis (Type A cases, which aligns with primary non-responsive CD), compared with individuals who experienced relapse of their symptoms after initial remission following a GFD (type B cases, which aligns with secondary non-responsive CD) [44]. Median time from index CD diagnosis to presentation with complications was 0.3 (0.1–1.4) years in Type A cases, compared with 4.9 (3.3–8.1) years in Type B cases [44] and overall mortality was higher in Type A cases compared with Type B cases (51% versus 25%) [44]. Moreover, homozygosity for HLA-DQ2 is present in a higher proportion of individuals with RCD I and RCD II, than those with uncomplicated CD (26% and 44% vs 21%, respectively) [8, 45]. This suggests that RCD and associated complications is more likely in older coeliac patients, those who present with primary non-responsiveness soon after their index CD diagnosis, HLA-DQ2 homozygous patients and those with persisting, or new, "alarm" symptoms. However, the absence of large datasets to base consensus guidelines on, coupled with the poor prognosis of individuals with RCD II and associated complications, suggests that clinicians should adopt a low threshold to perform both OGD and SBCE in those with non-responsive CD.

There is currently no consensus on the interval of endoscopic surveillance in established RCD; in the UK, experts recommend a 12-monthly interval of surveillance for patients with RCD I once treatment response is established and a 6-monthly interval for patients with RCD II [12]. Further studies are warranted to refine patient selection for SBCE and enteroscopy both for diagnosis and monitoring of RCD, to ensure cost, risk and caseload associated with endoscopy in RCD is appropriate.

Importantly, abdominal CT and MR studies, as well as CT or MR-enteroclysis, are important complementary investigations that may help to identify abnormal bowel wall thickening, SB tumours, or abdominal lymphadenopathy (Fig. 5) in

---

[2] Including abdominal pain, diarrhoea, weight loss, blood in faeces, faecal calprotectin elevation, or iron-deficiency anaemia [27].

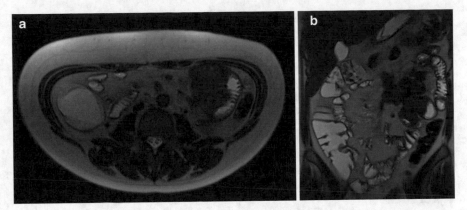

**Fig. 5** Transverse (**a**) and frontal (**b**) views of a magnetic resonance SB study in an individual with SB lymphoma. The images show a mesenteric mass with enlargement of adjacent nodes and a thickened proximal jejunal loop

individuals with suspected or established RCD/malignant complications [12]. In a study by Daum et al., detection of ulcerative jejunitis and EATL by capsule endoscopy, bi-directional endoscopy, abdominal CT and MR tomography were compared in 14 patients with RCD [46]. In one patient with RCD II, evidence of EATL was only identified by abdominal CT/MR tomography (as mesenteric lymphadenopathy) [46]. Indeed, EATL is often advanced at diagnosis and thus involves organs outside of the GI tract, so imaging studies are important to detect and stage malignant disease [3, 12]. In addition, cross-sectional imaging should also be considered when SBCE is contraindicated due to GI stenosis. However, imaging studies should not be undertaken at the expense of endoscopic assessment, as often mucosal lesions in RCD can be superficial and therefore, are more likely to be detected by direct mucosal inspection than on imaging studies alone [19].

## Conclusions

SBCE is a useful screening tool to assess individuals with suspicion for RCD, or established disease. It provides information regarding the presence of mucosal irregularities, extent of mucosal inflammation and helps to guide more invasive enteroscopy to obtain targeted biopsies. Imaging studies are important to complete the assessment of malignant complications and may be useful in those unable to undergo SBCE. Studies are needed to delineate the clinical, laboratory and endoscopic abnormalities associated with RCD and malignant complications, to improve case selection for more extensive small bowel endoscopic assessment.

**Supplementary Materials** None.

**Acknowledgements** No funding was obtained for this review. HAP is a Wellcome Clinical Fellow funded on grant 203,914/Z/16/Z to the Universities of Manchester, Leeds, Newcastle, and Sheffield. DSS receives an educational grant from Schaer (a gluten-free food manufacturer). Dr. Schaer did not have any input in drafting of this manuscript. Sheffield Teaching Hospitals NHS Trust is the NHS England National Centre for Refractory Coeliac Disease.

**Conflicts of Interest None.**

# References

1. Otuya DO, Verma Y, Farrokhi H, et al. Non-endoscopic biopsy techniques: a review. Expert Rev Gastroenterol Hepatol. 2018;12(2):109–17.
2. Vasile BD, Alina P, Mariana J. Chapter 6: novel endoscopic techniques in celiac disease. In: Rodrigo L, editor. Celiac disease and non-celiac gluten sensitivity. London, UK: IntechOpen; 2017.
3. Daveson AJ, Anderson RP. Small bowel endoscopy and coeliac disease. Best Pract Res Clin Gastroenterol. 2012;26(3):315–23.
4. Ludvigsson JF, Bai JC, Biagi F, et al. Diagnosis and management of adult coeliac disease: guidelines from the British Society of Gastroenterology. Gut. 2014;63(8):1210–28.
5. Chang MS, Rubin M, Lewis SK, Green PH. Diagnosing celiac disease by video capsule endoscopy (VCE) when esophagogastroduodenoscopy (EGD) and biopsy is unable to provide a diagnosis: a case series. BMC Gastroenterol. 2012;12:90.
6. Höroldt BS, ME MA, Stephenson TJ, Hadjivassiliou M, Sanders DS. Making the diagnosis of coeliac disease: is there a role for push enteroscopy? Eur J Gastroenterol Hepatol. 2004;16(11):1143.
7. Hopper AD, Cross SS, Sanders DS. Patchy villous atrophy in adult patients with suspected gluten-sensitive enteropathy: is a multiple duodenal biopsy strategy appropriate? Endoscopy. 2008;40(3):219–24.
8. Malamut G, Afchain P, Verkarre V, et al. Presentation and long-term follow-up of refractory celiac disease: comparison of type I with type II. Gastroenterology. 2009;136(1):81–90.
9. Roshan B, Leffler DA, Jamma S, et al. The incidence and clinical spectrum of refractory celiac disease in a North American referral center. Am J Gastroenterol. 2011;106(5):923–8.
10. Rowinski SA, Christensen E. Epidemiologic and therapeutic aspects of refractory coeliac disease - a systematic review. Dan Med J. 2016;63(12):A5307.
11. Ludvigsson JF, Leffler DA, Bai JC, et al. The Oslo definitions for coeliac disease and related terms. Gut. 2013;62(1):43–52.
12. Baggus EMR, Hadjivassiliou M, Cross S, et al. How to manage adult coeliac disease: perspective from the NHS England rare diseases collaborative network for non-responsive and refractory coeliac disease. Frontline Gastroenterol. 2019;11(3):235–42.
13. Cellier C, Patey N, Mauvieux L, et al. Abnormal intestinal intraepithelial lymphocytes in refractory sprue. Gastroenterology. 1998;114(3):471–81.
14. Lebwohl B, Kapel RC, Neugut AI, et al. Adherence to biopsy guidelines increases celiac disease diagnosis. Gastrointest Endosc. 2011;74:103–9.
15. Latorre M, Lagana SM, Freedberg DE, Lewis SK, Lebwohl B, Bhagat G, Green PHR. Endoscopic biopsy technique in the diagnosis of celiac disease: one bite or two? Gastrointest Endosc. 2015;81(5):1228–33.

16. Evans KE, Aziz I, Cross SS, et al. A prospective study of duodenal bulb biopsy in newly diagnosed and established adult celiac disease. Am J Gastroenterol. 2011;106:137–42.
17. Rubio-Tapia A, Kelly DG, Lahr BD, Dogan A, Wu TT, Murray JA. Clinical staging and survival in refractory celiac disease: a single center experience. Gastroenterology. 2009;136(1):99–107. quiz 352–103
18. Egan LJ, Walsh SV, Stevens FM, et al. Celiac-associated lymphoma. A single institution experience of 30 cases in the combination chemotherapy era. J Clin Gastroenterol. 1995;21(2):123–9.
19. Tomba C, Sidhu R, Sanders DS, et al. Celiac disease and double-balloon enteroscopy: what can we achieve? The experience of 2 European tertiary referral centers. J Clin Gastroenterol. 2016;50:313–7.
20. Zammit SC, Sanders DSS, Sidhu R. Capsule endoscopy for patients with coeliac disease. Expert Rev Gastroenterol Hepatol. 2018;12(8):779–90.
21. Barret M, Malamut G, Rahmi G, et al. Diagnostic yield of capsule endoscopy in refractory celiac disease. Am J Gastroenterol. 2012;107(10):1546–53.
22. Petroniene R, Dubcenco E, Baker JP, et al. Given capsule endoscopy in celiac disease: evaluation of diagnostic accuracy and interobserver agreement. Am J Gastroenterol. 2005;100:685–94.
23. Hopper AD, Sidhu R, Hurlstone DP, et al. Capsule endoscopy: an alternative to duodenal biopsy for the recognition of villous atrophy in coeliac disease? Dig Liver Dis. 2007;39:140–5.
24. Lidums I, Cummins AG, Teo E. The role of capsule endoscopy in suspected celiac disease patients with positive celiac serology. Dig Dis Sci. 2011;56:499–505.
25. Rondonotti E, Spada C, Cave D, et al. Video capsule enteroscopy in the diagnosis of celiac disease: a multicenter study. Am J Gastroenterol. 2007;102:1624–31.
26. Pennazio M, Spada C, Eliakim R, et al. Small-bowel capsule endoscopy and device-assisted enteroscopy for diagnosis and treatment of small bowel disorders: European Society of Gastrointestinal Endoscopy (ESGE) clinical guideline. Endoscopy. 2015;47:352–76.
27. Perez-Cuadrado-Robles E, Lujan-Sanchis M, Elli L, et al. Role of capsule endoscopy in alarm features and nonresponsive celiac disease: a European multicenter study. Dig Endosc. 2018;30:461–6.
28. Culliford A, Daly J, Diamond B, et al. The value of wireless capsule endoscopy in patients with complicated celiac disease. Gastrointest Endosc. 2005;62:55–61.
29. Atlas DS, Rubio-Tapia A, Van Dyke CT, et al. Capsule endoscopy in nonresponsive celiac disease. Gastrointest Endosc. 2011;74:1315–22.
30. Zammit SC, Sanders DS, Cross SS, Sidhu R. Capsule endoscopy in the management of refractory coeliac disease. J Gastrointestin Liver Dis. 2019;28:15–22.
31. Lidums I, Teo E, Field J, Adrian G, Cummins AG. Capsule endoscopy: a valuable tool in the follow-up of people with celiac disease on a gluten-free diet. Clin Transl Gastroenterol. 2011;2(8):e4.
32. Murray JA, Rubio-Tapia A, Van Dyke CT, et al. Mucosal atrophy in celiac disease: extent of involvement, correlation with clinical presentation, and response to treatment. Clin Gastroenterol Hepatol. 2008;6(2):186–93.
33. Liao Z, Gao R, Xu C, Li ZS. Indications and detection, completion, and retention rates of small-bowel capsule endoscopy: a systematic review. Gastrointest Endosc. 2010;71(2):280–6.
34. Pennazio M, Venezia L, Valdivia PC, et al. Device-assisted enteroscopy: an update on techniques, clinical indications and safety. Dig Liver Dis. 2019;51:934–43.
35. Cellier C, Cuillerier E, Patey-Mariaud de Serre N, et al. Push enteroscopy in celiac sprue and refractory sprue. Gastrointest Endosc. 1999;50(5):613–7.
36. Hadithi M, Al-Toma A, Oudejans J, et al. The value of double-balloon enteroscopy in patients with refractory celiac disease. Am J Gastroenterol. 2007;102(5):987–96.
37. Elli L, Casazza G, Locatelli M, et al. Use of enteroscopy for the detection of malignant and premalignant lesions of the small bowel in complicated celiac disease: a meta-analysis. Gastrointest Endosc. 2017;86(2):264–73.
38. Dewar DH, Donnelly SC, McLaughlin SD, Johnson MW, Ellis HJ, Ciclitira PJ. Celiac disease: management of persistent symptoms in patients on a gluten-free diet. World J Gastroenterol. 2012;18(12):1348–56.

39. Abdulkarim AS, Burgart LJ, See J, Murray JA. Etiology of nonresponsive celiac disease: results of a systematic approach. Am J Gastroenterol. 2002;97(8):2016–21.

40. Penny HA, Baggus EMR, Rej A, Snowden JA, Sanders DS. Non-responsive coeliac disease: a comprehensive review from the NHS England National Centre for refractory coeliac disease. Nutrients. 2020;12:216.

41. Leffler DA, Dennis M, Hyett B, et al. Etiologies and predictors of diagnosis in nonresponsive celiac disease. Clin Gastroenterol Hepatol. 2007;5:445–50.

42. Abdulkarim AS, Burgart LJ, See J, et al. Etiology of nonresponsive celiac disease: results of a systematic approach. Am J Gastroenterol. 2002;97:2016–21.

43. van Wanrooij RLJ, Bouma G, Bontkes HJ, et al. Outcome of referrals for non-responsive celiac disease in a tertiary center: low incidence of refractory celiac disease in the Netherlands. Clin Transl Gastroenterol. 2017;8:e218.

44. Biagi F, Marchese A, Ferretti F, et al. A multicentre case control study on complicated coeliac disease: two different patterns of natural history, two different prognoses. BMC Gastroenterol. 2014;14:139.

45. Al-Toma A, Goerres MS, Meijer JW, et al. Human leukocyte antigen-DQ2 homozygosity and the development of refractory celiac disease and enteropathy-associated T-cell lymphoma. Clin Gastroenterol Hepatol. 2006;4:315–9.

46. Daum S, Wahnschaffe U, Glasenapp R, et al. Capsule endoscopy in refractory celiac disease. Endoscopy. 2007;39(5):455–8.

# The Role of Pathologist in the Diagnosis of Refractory Coeliac Disease-and Enteropathy-Associated T Cell Lymphoma

Dominique Cazals-Hatem and Georgia Malamut

## Introduction

Histological examination of duodenal mucosa biopsies is the "gold standard" for diagnosis of coeliac disease (CD) in adults, based on a villous atrophy, crypt hyperplasia and a surface intraepithelial lymphocytosis. The recovery to a normal histology after at least 1 year of gluten-free diet (GFD) is the only way to confirm CD [1]. Persistent or recurring symptoms despite a strict GFD may announce a refractory coeliac disease (RCD) that needs complete re-evaluation of the disease including systematic review of initial and subsequent biopsies by an expert pathologist completed with immunohistochemistry, flow cytometry and molecular studies [2]. The hallmark lesions of CD are unspecific and may occur in other enteropathies or conditions. Additional upper and lower endoscopies with biopsies are required to exclude them and final diagnosis of RCD requires integration of standard histology, immunohistochemistry, clonality, serology and clinical data.

The pathologist has a major role in the characterisation of RCD and in follow-up to assess mucosal improvement after treatment. Morphological or phenotypic changes are interpreted in parallel with the monitoring of TCR clonality using the formalin-fixed paraffin-embedded mucosa (FFPE) samples for both analyses [3]. This approach improves early detection of neoplastic complications. Management of patients affected with RCD needs innovative therapies proposed by an expert

D. Cazals-Hatem (✉)
Department of Pathology, Beaujon Hospital AP-HP - University Paris France, Boulevard G Leclerc, Clichy, France
e-mail: dominique.cazals-hatem@aphp.fr

G. Malamut
Department of Gastroenterology, AP-HP. Centre-Université de Paris Hôpital Cochin, Paris, France
e-mail: georgia.malamut@aphp.fr

© Springer Nature Switzerland AG 2022
G. Malamut, N. Cerf-Bensussan (eds.), *Refractory Celiac Disease*,
https://doi.org/10.1007/978-3-030-90142-4_6

63

team to prevent transformation in enteropathy-associated T-cell lymphoma (EATL) which constitutes the most serious complication of CD.

## Refractory Coeliac Disease (RCD) Diagnosis

Refractory coeliac diseases (RCD) are defined as true CD which do not (primary resistance) or no longer respond to GFD (secondary resistance). In order to exclude inadvertent ingestion of gluten, RCD diagnosis requires negative coeliac serology and control by a dietitian of strict adherence to a GFD for more than 1 year [4]. Histological review by a skilled pathologist of the initial CD diagnosis together with evidence of a positive serology before GFD are prerequisite. Duodenal mucosal analysis requires at least four well-oriented biopsies from the second part of the duodenum to assess and compare accurately the villous architecture [1]. Normal duodenal histology with persistent clinical symptoms should lead to systematic colonic biopsies to discard microscopic colitis potentially associated to CD.

In the context of adequate GFD, RCD is defined histologically by the persistence of CD abnormalities namely a villous atrophy and an intraepithelial lymphocytosis. The villous atrophy is graded according to the modified Marsh-Oberhuber stage [5]. Pathologist assesses density of lymphocytosis by counting on H&E-stained sections at ×400 magnification the surface intraepithelial lymphocytes (IEL) per 100 enterocytes. Normal IEL are small lymphocytes with regular round nuclei, without nucleoli; the intra-epithelial lymphocytosis is homogeneous and intensified at the tips of villi if persistent. Hyperplasia of the crypts and diffuse lymphoplasmacytic infiltrate in the lamina propria are common; neutrophils and eosinophils are scarce but possibly observed in advanced stage disease [6]. The mucosal healing by GFD induces a complete recovery with normal villous architecture and a decrease of IEL [normal IEL count <30 IEL/100 epithelial cells in duodenum and <40 IEL/100 epithelial cells in jejunum (Marsh type 0)]. If villous atrophy and surface lymphocytosis persist, immunohistochemistry on FFPE sections is mandatory using the CD103, CD3, CD8, CD4, CD30 and granzyme B antibodies. The percentage of IEL labelled by each antibody must be correctly evaluated to conclude to a normal IEL phenotype defined by CD3 and CD8 coexpression in more than 60% of IEL with expression of CD103 without expression of CD30 and CD4 (IEL expressing CD4 < 10%). Normal IEL faintly express granzyme B.

Two types of RCD are recognized based on the surface immunophenotype of IEL and of TCR clonality analysis [2]. A normal IEL phenotype characterizes the RCD-type 1 (RCD1) and an abnormal IEL phenotype characterizes the RCD-type 2 (RCD2). This differentiation by the pathologist is fundamental for patient management since the prognosis is radically different [7], RCD2 being considered as an intestinal low grade lymphoma.

## Type 1 RCD (RCD1)

In RCD1, the duodenal mucosa shows villous atrophy (Marsh type 3) and a diffuse increase in IEL that is strictly identical to that observed in untreated and uncomplicated CD. Villous atrophy may be patchy or variable among specimens and the surface lymphocytosis is generally marked made of normal-looking lymphocytes that display a normal phenotype CD103+, CD3+, CD8+, CD4−, CD30− (Fig. 1).

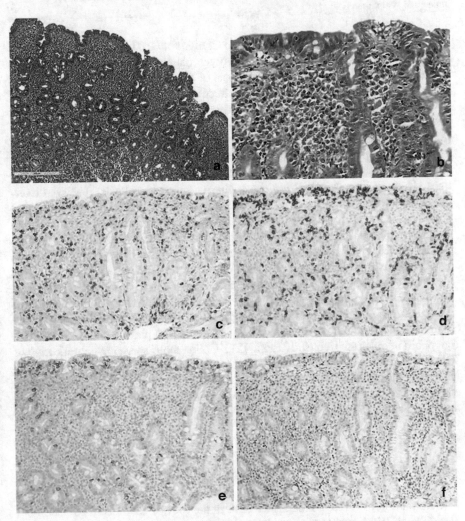

**Fig. 1** Refractory coeliac disease type 1 (RCD1) in a duodenal paraffin-embedded biopsy. (**a** and **b**) The villous atrophy is total (Marsh type 3) and intraepithelial lymphocytes (IEL) are increased (>40/100 enterocytes) in the surface epithelium with numerous plama cells well-seen in lamina propria. (**c**) IEL express CD3. (**d**) all IEL express CD8. (**e**) all IEL express CD103. (**f**) IEL faintly express granzyme B

**Table 1** Conditions or diseases mimicking coeliac enteropathy

Infectious, viral enteritis—tropical sprue
Bacterial overgrowth syndrome
Crohn's disease
Eosinophilic gastroenteritis
Radiation-induced or ischemic enteritis
Common variable immunodeficiency, IgA deficiency
Autoimmune enteritis
Drug effects (olmesartan, mycophenolate, azathioprine, methotrexate, chemotherapy)
Intestinal lymphoma

The proportion of IEL expressing CD3 and CD8 is above 60 percent. The TCR gene rearrangement analysis by PCR shows a polyclonal profile.

However, the RCD1 remains a diagnosis of exclusion after discarding all non-CD enteropathies displaying villous architectural changes (Table 1). Histological features atypical for a classic CD or indicative of other etiologies have to be searched and reported specially in seronegative enteropathy with primary resistance to GFD [8]. In case of secondary resistance, additional conditions could interfere in producing villous atrophy and / or lymphocytosis. Histologically, surface lymphocytosis without villous atrophy (Marsh type 1 or 2) could suggest chronic intestinal infections (*Helicobacter pylori*, *Giardia intestinalis*, microsporidiosis), bacterial overgrowth or Crohn's disease that needs further investigations (capsule endoscopy and ileal biopsies…) [9]. Chronic ischemia and radiation-induced enteritis generate crypt atrophy and interstitial fibrosis. Distinctive features such as diffuse neutrophilic, eosinophilic, granulomatous infiltrates, cryptitis or crypt necrosis, basal crypt apoptosis, yield specific clues for differential diagnoses (Fig. 2). Both the olmesartan-induced enteropathy and the exceptional autoimmune enteropathy display numerous apoptotic bodies at the base of crypts and also have close clinical and biological presentation [10]. Lamina propria in enteropathy associated with common variable immune deficiency (CIVD) is devoid of plasma cells and reactive lymphoid nodules are frequently found [11]. Collagenous sprue is a complication of CD that is often associated with RCDI: it is characterized by subepithelial deposition of a collagen band thicker than 15 μm highlighted by trichrome or sirius stains (Fig. 2) [12]. The physiopathology of such deposition is still unknown and denotes advanced stage disease.

## Type 2 RCD (RCD2)

For the pathologist, the hallmark of RCD2 is the loss of CD8 expression in more than 50% of IEL interpreted as an abnormal (aberrant) phenotype. A routine FFPE-based immunohistochemistry using the panel—CD103, CD3, CD8, CD4, CD30 and granzyme B—is the simplest method to confirm the abnormal loss of T-cell surface antigens (CD3, CD8, TCR) with maintain of normal intracellular expression of CD3. The exact number of IEL with aberrant phenotype (i.e. CD103+CD3+CD8−CD4−) must be carefully counted to confirm the emergence of an abnormal IEL

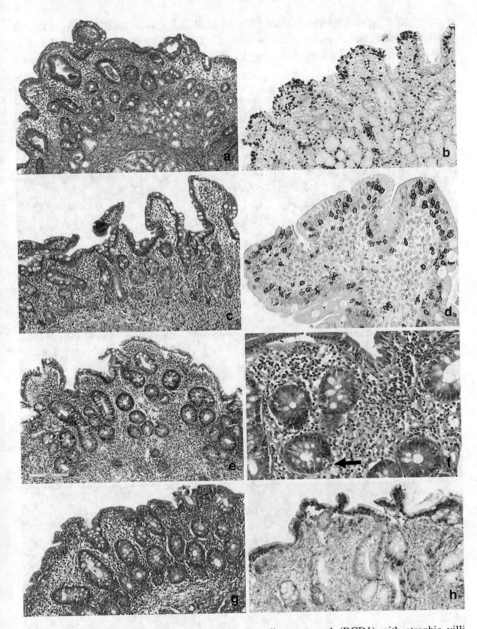

**Fig. 2** Enteropathies mimicking refractory cocliac disease type 1 (RCD1) with atrophic villi (Marsh type 3) in duodenal paraffin-embedded biopsies, immunostained with CD8 antibody. (**a** and **b**) Chronic duodenitis associated with *Helicobacter pilori* infection in coeliac disease: patchy villous atrophy combined to accumulation of CD8+ intraepithelial lymphocytes (IEL) in the villi's dome may mimick RCD1. (**c** and **d**) Olmesartan-induced enteropathy gives various villous atrophy with a significant increase of CD8+ IEL. (**e** and **f**) Common variable immune deficiency-associated enteropathy presented with subtotal villous atrophy and interstital polymorphous inflammation in lamina propria devoid of plasma cells revealing hypogammaglobulinemia; apototic bodies in basal cell crypts are well-seen (arrow). (**g** and **h**) Collagen sprue secondarily observed in a coeliac disease display a red collagene band beneath the surface epithelium stained by sirius-hemalun combined with total villous atrophy and and large increase of CD8+ IEL

population representing more than 50% of total IEL CD103+CD3+. Thus RCD2 diagnosis relies on the association of villous atrophy (Marsh type 3, Figs. 3 and 4) with detection of aberrant IEL by FFPE immunohistochemistry or by flow

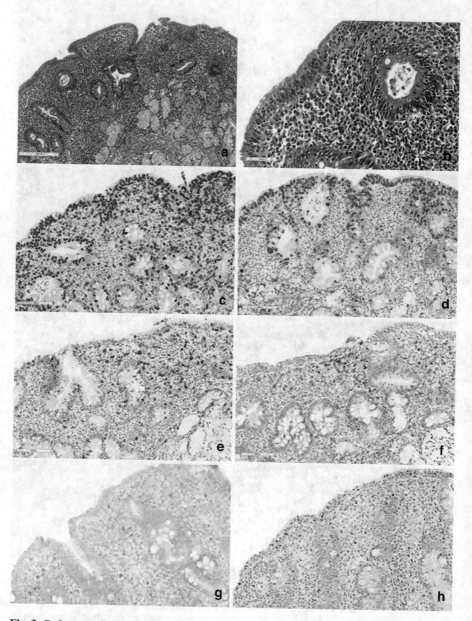

**Fig. 3** Refractory coeliac disease type 2 (RCD2) in a duodenal paraffin-embedded biopsy. (**a** and **b**) The villous atrophy is total (Marsh type 3) and intraepithelial lymphocytosis is marked and diffuse, made of homogenous normal-looking small lymphocytes. (**c**) CD3+ intraepithelial lymphocytes (IEL) are increased in the surface epithelium. (**d**) IEL express CD103. (**e**) Less than 50% of IEL express CD8 indicating an aberrant abnormal phenotype. (**f**) No IEL express CD4. (**g**) No IEL express CD30. (**h**) IEL faintly express granzyme B

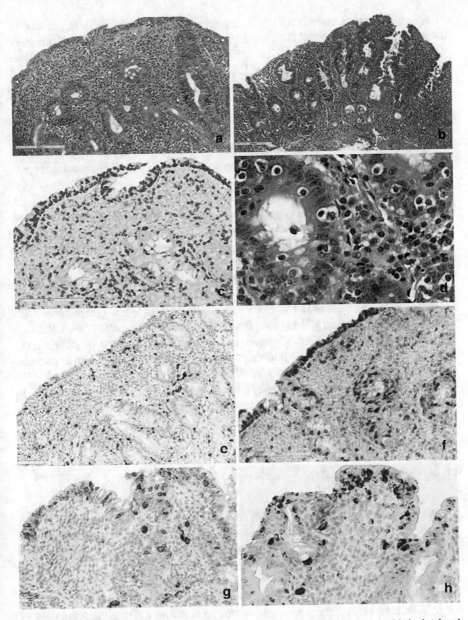

**Fig. 4** Refractory coeliac disease type 2 (RCD2) complicated with ulcerative jejunitis in duodenal paraffin-embedded biopsies. (**a** and **b**) The villous atrophy is total and a tendancy to glandular distorsion and interstitial fibrosis is observed. (**c**) CD3+ intraepithelial lymphocytes (IEL) are increased in the surface epithelium. (**d**) Some IEL in halot shows irregular nuclear contour and nucleoli. (**e**) Less than 50% of IEL express CD8 indicating an aberrant abnormal phenotype. (**f**) IEL express CD103. (**g**) IEL express diffusely CD30. (**h**) Granzyme B is highly expressed in all IEL

cytometry. The latter technique, which requires fresh tissue, is necessary to detect low percentages of abnormal IEL, as much more sensible to identify small numbers of IEL expressing cytoplasmic CD3 without surface CD3 [7]. It is also useful to identify rare cases in which abnormal IEL express CD8.

According to a recent CELAC group study [13], the expression of NKp46 antibody (NK-receptor antibody applicable on FFPE tissue) in more than 25 IEL per 100 enterocytes looks determinant to differentiate the RCD1 to RCD2; its use in routine could be generalized meanwhile waiting for molecular TCR analysis. Expression of CD30 by many aberrant IEL must lead to fear transformation into high grade lymphoma [14] and a high expression of granzyme B is associated (personal data).

In addition to histological data, analysis of TCR rearrangements by PCR on DNA extracted from mucosal biopsies (frozen or FFPE) is fundamental to confirm RCD2 diagnosis: it generally shows a monoclonal profile but oligoclonal rearrangement is not exclusive of RCD2 diagnosis [7]. Even if aberrant IEL displays a normal morphology, the RCD2 stage corresponds genetically to the emergence of a malignant *in-situ* clone equivalent to an intra-epithelial T-cell lymphoma, requiring intensive therapy.

RCD2 must be differentiated from other intestinal indolent lymphomas with TCR rearrangements and villous atrophy. Indeed, the intestinal CD4 or CD8 T-cell indolent lymphomas may cause lymphomatous epitheliotropism with villous atrophy but T-cell infiltration of the lamina propria is manifest on immunohistochemistry [15]. Exceptional observations of CD57+ T-cell large granular lymphocyte leukemia localized in small bowel may be very tricky to differentiate from RCD2 in a coeliac patient, overall recalling the importance of a multidisciplinary approach to discard all other causes of enteropathy [16].

## Ulcerative Jejunoileitis

Some patients with RCD2 present with concomitant ulcerative jejunoileitis conferring a worse prognosis due to malnutrition associated with protein loss enteropathy. During follow-up of subsequent duodenal exulceration, glandular distortion and interstitial fibrosis are highly indicative of pejorative evolution and exhort to further investigations to detect ulcer, nodules, plaques, strictures or nodules in jejunum or ileum. Because of superimposed acute inflammation, these manifestations may be tricky to interpret and require generous sampling to isolate infiltrating aggregates of aberrant IEL (CD3+ CD103+ CD8−) with upregulated cytotoxic content revealed by strong granzyme B expression. The presence of IEL with atypical features—i.e. heterogeneous in shape or size with irregular contour larger nuclei and nucleoli and expressing CD30—is the clue for proposing lymphoma transformation (Fig. 4) [14]. The diagnostic difficulty for pathologists is to evoke an ulcerative jejunitis in first inaugural manifestations of CD; intestinal biopsies done in more distal parts of the small intestine help to suggest a latent or complicated CD and ultimately TCR clonality confirms underlying RDC2 [7].

## Enteropathy-Associated T-Cell Lymphoma (EATL)

In established CD, the pathologist has no difficulty to recognize overt EATL that presents as massive parietal infiltration of lymphoma T-cells in the jejunum or the ileum. Moreover, many cases are complicated by perforation. Colonic and gastric locations are uncommon and inaugural extra-gastrointestinal presentations are exceptional (skin, liver, nervous system) [17]. Lymphoma cells are typically pleo-morphic, medium to large, with vesicular multinucleated nuclei, prominent nucleoli and a frequent anaplastic morphology. Eosinophils, apoptotic cells and necrosis are current mixed with angioinvasion features. In surgical small bowel resection, mes-enteric lymph nodes show intrasinusal infiltration, necrosis or degenerative cavita-tion [17].

The non-involved mucosa far or adjacent to ulcers generally shows villous atro-phy and intraepithelial lymphocytosis indicative of concomitant CD or RCD2 when IEL display an aberrant phenotype identical to lymphoma cells. The immunopheno-type of EATL cells classically is CD3+, CD103+, CD30+, granzyme B+, CD8−, CD4−, CD5−, CD56− (Fig. 5). The CD8 may be expressed in "de novo" EATL without prior RCD2 [18]. EBV is always absent. In case of unknown CD, diffuse expression of CD103 is fundamental to propose EATL [17]. Differential diagnoses are the anaplastic large T-cell lymphoma (ALK1+) and the aggressive extranodal NK/T cell lymphoma occasionally localized to the intestine with similar cytotoxic activity but EBV is often detected in lymphoma cells [19].

## Conclusion

The pathologist plays an fundamental role in RCD diagnosis in order to exclude other enteropathies, to characterize the type of RCD and to monitor mucosal healing of patients under adapted treatment. Specific immunohistochemical markers are necessary to identify the type of RCD and to eliminate other indolent intestinal lymphoproliferative disorders. Monitoring morphological changes ie resolution versus worsening of villous atrophy is indispensable to adapt therapy and to estab-lish prognosis. Progression to overt EATL is rare but dramatic and all disciplines and strategies must cooperate for early detection and rapid access to intensive ther-apy in order to improve prognosis.

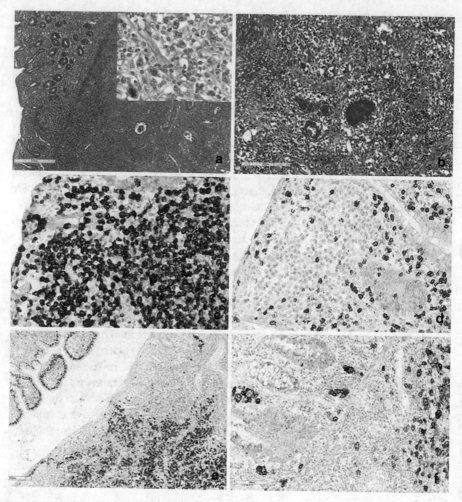

**Fig. 5** Enteropathy-associated T-cell lymphoma complicated with ileal perforation in a surgical resection specimen. (**a** and **b**) The parietal infiltration by pleomorphic medium to large lymphoma cells (insert) is mixed with inflammatory cells and necrosis increased by angioinvasion and microthrombosis. (**c**) In the lamina propria, small to medium lymphoma cells express CD3. (**d**) the lymphoma cells expressing CD3 do not express CD8. (**e**) Lymphoma cells express CD103, as the intraepithelial lymphocytosis does in preserved ileal mucosa seen in the upper left corner. (**f**) Anaplastic lymphoma cells invading the lymphatic vessels express CD30

## References

1. Lebwohl B, Rubio-Tapia A. Epidemiology, presentation, and diagnosis of celiac disease. Gastroenterology. 2021;160(1):63–75.
2. Malamut G, Cellier C. Refractory celiac disease. Gastroenterol Clin North Am. 2019;48(1):137–44.

3. Derrieux C, Trinquand A, Bruneau J, Verkarre V, Lhermitte L, Alcantara M, et al. A single-tube, EuroClonality-inspired, TRG clonality multiplex PCR aids management of patients with enteropathic diseases, including from formaldehyde-fixed, paraffin-embedded tissues. J Mol Diagn. 2019;21(1):111–22.
4. Rubio-Tapia A, Hill ID, Kelly CP, Calderwood AH, Murray JA, American College of Gastroenterology. ACG clinical guidelines: diagnosis and management of celiac disease. Am J Gastroenterol. 2013;108(5):656–76. quiz 677
5. Oberhuber G, Granditsch G, Vogelsang H. The histopathology of coeliac disease: time for a standardized report scheme for pathologists. Eur J Gastroenterol Hepatol. 1999;11(10):1185–94.
6. Brown IS, Smith J, Rosty C. Gastrointestinal pathology in celiac disease: a case series of 150 consecutive newly diagnosed patients. Am J Clin Pathol. 2012;138(1):42–9.
7. Malamut G, Afchain P, Verkarre V, Lecomte T, Amiot A, Damotte D, et al. Presentation and long-term follow-up of refractory celiac disease: comparison of type I with type II. Gastroenterology. 2009;136(1):81–90.
8. Leonard MM, Lebwohl B, Rubio-Tapia A, Biagi F. AGA clinical practice update on the evaluation and management of seronegative enteropathies: expert review. Gastroenterology. 2021;160(1):437–44.
9. Lauwers GY, Fasano A, Brown IS. Duodenal lymphocytosis with no or minimal enteropathy: much ado about nothing? Mod Pathol. 2015;28 Suppl 1:S22–9.
10. Scialom S, Malamut G, Meresse B, Guegan N, Brousse N, Verkarre V, et al. Gastrointestinal disorder associated with olmesartan mimics autoimmune enteropathy. PLoS One. 2015;10(6):e0125024.
11. Malamut G, Verkarre V, Suarez F, Viallard J-F, Lascaux A-S, Cosnes J, et al. The enteropathy associated with common variable immunodeficiency: the delineated frontiers with celiac disease. Am J Gastroenterol. 2010;105(10):2262–75.
12. Rubio-Tapia A, Talley NJ, Gurudu SR, Wu T-T, Murray JA. Gluten-free diet and steroid treatment are effective therapy for most patients with collagenous sprue. Clin Gastroenterol Hepatol. 2010;8(4):344–9.e3.
13. Cheminant M, Bruneau J, Malamut G, Sibon D, Guegan N, van Gils T, et al. NKp46 is a diagnostic biomarker and may be a therapeutic target in gastrointestinal T-cell lymphoproliferative diseases: a CELAC study. Gut. 2019;68(8):1396–405.
14. Farstad IN, Johansen F-E, Vlatkovic L, Jahnsen J, Scott H, Fausa O, et al. Heterogeneity of intracpithelial lymphocytes in refractory sprue: potential implications of CD30 expression. Gut. 2002;51(3):372–8.
15. Malamut G, Meresse B, Kaltenbach S, Derrieux C, Verkarre V, Macintyre E, et al. Small intestinal CD4+ T-cell lymphoma is a heterogenous entity with common pathology features. Clin Gastroenterol Hepatol. 2014;12(4):599–608.e1.
16. Malamut G, Meresse B, Verkarre V, Kaltenbach S, Montcuquet N, Duong Van Huyen J-P, et al. Large granular lymphocytic leukemia: a treatable form of refractory celiac disease. Gastroenterology. 2012;143(6):1470–72.e2.
17. Swerdlow SH, Campo E, Pileri SA, Harris NL, Stein H, Siebert R, et al. The 2016 revision of the World Health Organization classification of lymphoid neoplasms. Blood. 2016;127(20):2375–90.
18. Malamut G, Chandesris O, Verkarre V, Meresse B, Callens C, Macintyre E, et al. Enteropathy associated T cell lymphoma in celiac disease: a large retrospective study. Dig Liver Dis. 2013;45(5):377–84.
19. van Vliet C, Spagnolo DV. T- and NK-cell lymphoproliferative disorders of the gastrointestinal tract: review and update. Pathology (Phila). 2020;52(1):128–41.

# Laboratory Findings for the Diagnosis of Celiac Disease Related Complications

Chantal Brouzes, Sascha Cording, Amel Bensalah, Vahid Asnafi, Nadine Cerf-Bensussan, and Ludovic Lhermitte

## Abbreviations

| | |
|---|---|
| CD | Celiac disease |
| cy | Cytoplasmic |
| EATL | Enteropathy Associated T-cell lymphoma |
| GFD | Gluten-free diet |
| i | Intracellular |
| IEL | Intra-Epithelial Lymphocytes |
| LGL | Large Granular Lymphocytes |
| LPL | Lamina Propria Lymphocytes |
| RCD | Refractory celiac disease |
| sm | Surface membrane |
| TCR | T-cell receptor |

C. Brouzes · A. Bensalah
Laboratory of Onco-Haematology, AP-HP, Hôpital Necker Enfants-Malades, Paris, France

S. Cording
Université de Paris, Imagine Institute, Laboratory of Intestinal Immunity, INSERM UMR1163, Paris, France

V. Asnafi · L. Lhermitte (✉)
Laboratory of Onco-Haematology, AP-HP, Hôpital Necker Enfants-Malades, Paris, France

Université de Paris, Institut Necker-Enfants-Malades, INSERM UMR 1151, Paris, France
e-mail: vahid.asnafi@aphp.fr; ludovic.lhermitte@aphp.fr

N. Cerf-Bensussan
Laboratory of Intestinal Immunity, Université de Paris, INSERM UMR 1163 and Imagine Institute, Paris, France

© Springer Nature Switzerland AG 2022
G. Malamut, N. Cerf-Bensussan (eds.), *Refractory Celiac Disease*,
https://doi.org/10.1007/978-3-030-90142-4_7

# Introduction

Celiac disease (CeD) is a common chronic immune disorder characterized by a gluten-induced enteropathy in genetically predisposed individuals [1, 2]. A gluten-free diet (GFD) is usually an effective treatment, which resolves symptoms and enables histological recovery within less than 2 years. However, a small subset of patients experience persisting or recurring symptoms despite strict adherence to GFD and absence of other concomitant intestinal diseases. Non-responsive CeD with no obvious etiology are diagnosed with refractory-celiac disease (RCD) [3–6]. Two entities are currently recognized, type I (RCDI) and type II (RCDII), based on immunophenotypic and molecular features of the intraepithelial lymphocytes (IELs). RCDI is characterized by a polyclonal accumulation of IELs displaying a normal immunophenotype, while RCDII represents a clonal proliferation of immunophenotypically "aberrant" IELs. As such, RCDII can be defined as a 'cryptic' or low-grade 'intraepithelial' lymphoma, and represents a rare condition at high risk of transformation into overt and aggressive enteropathy-associated lymphoma (EATL) in up to 50% within 5 years [7–12]. RCDII and EATL share a similar clonal expansion of abnormal IELs, but they differ in the aspect that RCDII is characterized by the accumulation of non-proliferative small CD30− IELs while EATL shows aggressive features with the expansion of highly proliferative CD30+ large cells [13]. Altogether, CeD-related lymphomas encompass a heterogeneous group of disorders characterized by loss of homeostasis, which is a hallmark in cancer. Even though they represent a continuum certainly reflecting a stepwise oncogenic process, they bear distinctive characteristics with clinical significance. Precise identification of the different entities is of utmost importance as RCDI and RCDII benefit from distinct treatment approaches and RCDII but not RCDI bear a high risk of transformation into EATL. Diagnosis of EATL and its distinction from RCDII is also critical; Thus, RCDII results from the accumulation of slow-dividing cells that poorly respond to chemotherapy and chemotherapy may promote and accelerate the transformation of RCDII into overt EATL. Conversely, EATL represents the expansion of actively dividing cells and requires other treatment strategies including chemotherapy and hematopoietic stem-cell transplantation [14]. Finally it is important to define whether EATL complicates or not RCDII as prognosis of EATL complicating RCDII is much worse than if developing in patients with CD or RCDI (see chapter by Cording et al. mechanisms of lymphomagenesis).

Diagnosis of these entities relies on a body of evidence including histopathological and laboratory findings. In this chapter, we describe the laboratory tools routinely used to detect and characterize CeD-related lymphomas and provide clinically relevant guidance. Histopathological features are described in the chapter by Cazal-Hatem et al. HLA-typing and serum anti-transglutaminase antibodies are essential for the diagnosis of CeD but do not strictly represent an integral part of the diagnosis of CeD-related lymphomas. Herein, we describe the phenotypic and molecular features of intestinal lymphocytes in RCDI, RCDII and EATL, and discuss how they help to precisely characterize the disease. Recent advances in the understanding of CeD and its complications suggest that CeD-related lymphomas result from the acquisition of genetic events that drive cell-autonomous expansion of clonal intraepithelial cells. Diagnostic strategies take advantage of this phenomenon to properly identify quantitative changes in the distribution of the lymphoid resident cells, abnormal cell immunophenotypes, and clonality in the small intestinal tissue.

## Immunophenotypic Characteristics

### Phenotypical Characteristics of Intestinal Lymphocytes in the Normal Human Intestine, in CD and in RCD. Application for Diagnosis by Flow Cytometry

The small intestine is one of the richest tissues in lymphoid cells. Distinct populations of resident lymphoid cells distribute within the epithelium (IELs) and lamina propria. In the normal adult human intestine, IELs are mainly T cells. Approximately, 75% are CD8+ TCRαβ+ T-cells, 5–10% are CD4+ TCRαβ+ T-cells and 10–20% are TCRγδ T-cells. CD8+ TCRαβ+ T-IELs resemble circulating antigen-experienced T-cells: they express intracellular (i) CD3, and surface (sm) CD3, as well as CD7 and CD2 antigens but display variable CD5 expression [15, 16]. TCRγδ+ IELs express smCD3, iCD3, CD7, and CD2. They lack CD5, CD4 and generally CD8 although some can express CD8α. A minor subset (approximately 2–15% of IELs) consists of innate lymphoid cells (ILCs), that do not express surface TCR, CD3 or CD5 but show bright CD7 expression. In addition to NKG2D that they share with CD8+ TCRαβ+ and TCRγδ+ -IELs, they variably express several NK receptors, notably NPK44 and NKP46 [17]. A small fraction (20–30%) contains iCD3. All IELs, including ILCs, express CD103, the αE integrin subunit that associates with β7 integrin and promotes their local retention via binding to epithelial E-cadherin. In contrast, dominant cell subsets in the normal lamina propria, are IgA plasma cells and CD4+ TCRαβ+ lymphocytes (~60–70% of T cells) that comprise a variety of subsets including 5–15% of regulatory T-cells.

Active CD is characterized by a massive expansion of CD8+ TCRαβ+ IELs. As a consequence, the proportion of TCRγδ+ IELs and of ILC-like IELs tend to decrease. Following GFD, the absolute number of CD8+ TCRαβ+ IELs decreases while that of TCRγδ+ IELs tend to increase, so that the proportion of the latter cells can reach over 30% of all IELs [18, 19]. IgA plasma cells expand in the lamina propria during active CD. As they cannot be easily extracted from intestinal biopsies for flow cytometry analysis, they will not be discussed further and we will focus on the phenotypic characteristics IEL which are useful for differential diagnosis between CD, RCDI on one hand and RCDII on the other hand.

In RCDI, the phenotype of IEL remains comparable to that observed in CD, i.e. dominated by CD8+TCRαβ+ T cells. In keeping with the fact that patients are on GFD, an increased proportion of TCRγδ+ IEL (>30%) can be observed. In our experience, some patients can also display a small excess of CD4+ TCRαβ+ T-cells (15–20%).

In RCDII, the absolute number of IELs is increased and often more than in active CD or in RCDI. Yet, in contrast with CD and RCDI, the IELs that expand are, in the vast majority of patients, not T cells but innate-like IELs with an unusual and characteristic phenotype. Typically, RCDII IELs are CD103+ lymphocytes that lack surface expression of CD3 (smCD3−) and of T cell receptor (smTCR−) but which, unexpectedly, display massive intracellular expression of CD3 (iCD3). They are CD7+ but CD5− CD127− CD56− CD8−. They express CD122 (IL-2/15Rβ), NK receptors and notably NKG2D and NK46 and usually contain granzyme B, a cytotoxic marker (Fig. 1) [19–21]. In RCDII, the proportion of iC3+ ILC-like IEL is variable, generally between 50 and 95%. Yet it can be less in some patients and a threshold of 20% of iC3+ IELs is considered sufficient for the diagnosis of RCDII. As discussed in the chapter by Cording et al., the unusual phenotype of RCDII IELs has recently been ascribed to their origin from the very small sub-subset of ILC-like IELs that contain intracellular CD3 (see above). As discussed by Cording et al. and below, these cells have acquire gain-of function somatic mutations in the JAK-STAT pathway that licence their clonal expansion and cytolytic activation in the cytokine-rich environment of the celiac intestine. Of note, RCDII cells can extend into lamina propria, where their frequency remains however lower than in IELs, and also in blood or other tissues [22, 23]. Their expression of CD103 and their characteristic phenotype allow for their precise tracking.

While virtually all RCDII arise from a transformed clone of innate-like T-IELs, there are some exceptions. In rare RCDII cases, the clonal intraepithelial lymphoproliferation develops from CD103+ TCRγδ+ or even from TCRαβ+ IELs with possible expression of CD8 and/or NKP46.

EATL share the same clonal origin as RCDII and thereby share most immunological features. Yet, their highly malignant nature is attested by the increased size and abnormal cytology of the cells, their frequent expression of the activation marker CD30 and their high proliferative turnover rate as attested by the expression of the proliferation marker Ki67. In contrast to RCDII, EATL is generally a localized proliferation that can arise in all parts of the small intestine or sometimes in the mesenteric lymph nodes, more rarely at sites distant from intestine. Although some immunophenotypic features may be identified by flow cytometry, they are not sufficient for the diagnosis of EATL which relies on histological and immunohistochemical criteria (see the chapter by Cazals-Hatem et al). Yet, flow cytometry analysis of lymphocytes isolated from duodenum of patients with EATL is useful to define whether EATL complicates RCDII or arises de novo. Indeed, as discussed in the chapter by Cording et al., prognosis of EATL complicating RCDII is even more severe than that of EATL arising de novo in CD or RCDI (0% versus 50% of survival at 5 years respectively).

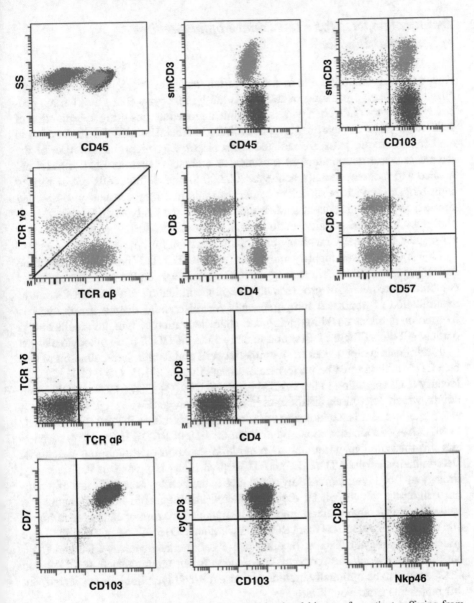

**Fig. 1** Immunophenotypic aspect of IEL from the duodenal biopsy of a patient suffering from RCDII. Green events represent smCD3+ cells from the immune microenvironment. Orange events represent the expanded compartment of ILCs which demonstrate qualitative aberrancies on top of quantitative increase. ILCs from this patient are smCD3− CD7+ CD103+ iCD3+ CD8− Nkp46+ and exceed 20% of CD45+ cells

# Technical Aspects for Flow Immunophenotyping of Duodenal Biopsies

Flow cytometry requires cells in suspension for analysis. Protocols have been optimized for selective isolation of intraepithelial lymphocytes (IEL) and lamina propria lymphocytes (LPL) in a two-step technical procedure, resulting in separation of cells from these compartments and avoiding artificial alterations in membrane marker expression. IELs are isolated from biopsies by vigorous agitation of the sample at warm temperature in presence of a chelator such as EDTA. Cells are washed and recovery usually achieves 200,000 to one million cells out of four to eight biopsies, which is sufficient to perform minimal flow cytometry assays and consider eventual subsequent studies such as molecular analysis on separated lymphocytes or cryopreservation of intestinal lymphocytes. LPLs are extracted by a subsequent step usually involving enzymatic digestion for lymphocyte release.

Flow cytometry can identify and quantify the RCDII ILC-like cells to determine their (ab)normal nature. There is no definitive consensus on the minimal antibody-combination required for proper analysis and identification of RCDII ILCs and/or identification of abnormal lymphoid cells for differential diagnosis. Analysis is focused on antigens enabling gating and characterization of lymphoid cells and in particular T-cells (Table 1). Staining must include the CD45 pan-leukocyte antigen to discriminate lymphocytes from epithelial cells and debris. Intracellular and surface CD3 staining must be performed associated with CD103, CD7, CD4, CD8 to identify ILCs according to the smCD3− cyCD3 CD103+ CD7+ CD4− CD8− phenotype which determines an aberrant immunophenotype (Fig. 1). Quantification is also important as it is a diagnostic criterion with at least 20% iCD3+ ILC-like cells in RCDII. Aside identification and characterization of RCDII IELs, some parameters are measured in particular to provide clues about a differential diagnosis. Determination of the CD4/CD8 and TCRαβ/γδ ratios is pivotal in the screening strategy of T-cell lymphomas. Any unbalance in these ratios is an indicator of potential lymphoma which can be then deciphered using specific immunophenotypic strategies. Some other markers may also be included for further characterization of other lymphoproliferation than RCDII, including CD16, CD56, CD57 for large granular lymphocytes disease, or other pan-T cell markers such as CD2 and CD5, but this falls beyond the scope of this review. B-cell markers such as CD19 and CD20 may also be optionally included in case a B-cell lymphoma is suspected, but this represents a rare condition.

# Value of Flow-Cytometry in the Diagnostic Work-Up: Advantages and Limitations

Diagnosis of RCDII benefits from a multidisciplinary approach and flow cytometry represents one piece of the diagnostic work-up. Each analytical tool provides complementary evidence and has advantages and limitations. Flow cytometry is a

**Table 1** Relevant antigens for immunophenotyping of lymphocytes from the gut tissue

| | |
|---|---|
| CD45 | **Panleukocyte antigen**<br>This antigen is present on all nucleated leukocytes including lymphocytes and allows accurate discrimination between lymphocytes and red cells, epithelial cells and debris.<br>This marker is essential for the gating strategy and represents the first step before dissection of the lymphocytes subsets. |
| CD3 | **Signaling component of the TCR complex**<br>This molecule is expressed by all mature and functional T-cells regardless the TCR type ($\alpha\beta$, $\gamma\delta$).<br>This marker is essential to separate the analysis along with the smCD3+ and smCD3− dichotomy. Exploration of smCD3+ cells allows for the characterization of normal resident lymphoid T-cells and the evaluation of the distribution of the distinct subsets (CD4/CD8, TCR$\alpha\beta$/TCR$\gamma\delta$) so that an eventual non-RCDII lymphoproliferation may be screened. Exploration of smCD3− cells allows identification and characterization of ILCs, and eventually of other lymphocytes subsets (B and NK-cells).<br>In addition, CD3 may be present in the cytoplasm although not expressed at the surface membrane in non-TCR expressing lymphoid cells (NK cells, ILCs).<br>Analysis of cyCD3 (or iCD) expression represents a major criteria for evaluation of ILC physiological diversity in clinics and is used as a criteria for abnormality when massively expressed (loss of diversity). |
| CD4<br>CD8 | **Receptor for the CMH I (CD8) and II (CD4) molecules**<br>These molecules are present on T-lymphocytes subsets. CD8 may also be expressed on other subsets such as NK cells.<br>These markers are useful to investigate distribution on T-cells in the gut in order to screen unbalances in their distribution calling for mature T-cell lymphoma with a gut infiltration.<br>CD8 is also useful for the characterization of ILCs which do not express CD8.<br>Absence of expression of CD8 on expanded ILCs supports a diagnosis of RCDII (although it may be expressed on rare occasions (<5%)) by contrast to some other mature T-cell lymphoproliferations. |
| TCR$\alpha\beta$<br>TCR$\gamma\delta$ | **T-cell receptors**<br>These molecules are expressed by all normal mature T-cells in a mutually exclusive manner.<br>These markers are useful to investigate distribution on T-cells in the gut in order to screen unbalances in their distribution calling for mature T-cell lymphoma with an infiltration of the intestine. |
| CD16<br>CD56<br>CD57<br>Granzyme B<br>Perforin<br>Nkp46 | **Cytotoxic molecules**<br>These molecules are broadly expressed by cytotoxic cells including NK and CD8+ T-cells.<br>These markers are useful as hallmarks of cytotoxic activity. They may help in determining the cytotoxic nature of a NK or T-cell expansion calling for a possible LGL disease.<br>Granzym B may also be helpful in characterization of ILCs, as well as Nkp46 to identify distinctive features of abnormal ILCs. |

(continued)

**Table 1** (continued)

| CD7 CD2 CD5 | **Pan-T cell antigens** These molecules are expressed by all mature T-cells. NK cells are also CD2+ and CD7+ but CD5−. ILCs are constantly CD7+ whenever normal, reactive or malignant. These markers are useful for characterization of mature T-cells. Any loss of a pan-T cell markers calls to a potential mature T-cell lymphoma. CD7 is also an essential marker to identify ILCs characterized by the smCD3− CD7+ CD103+ immunophenotype. |
|---|---|
| CD103 | **αE integrin** This molecule is broadly expressed on gut lymphocytes while virtually absent from circulating lymphocytes. CD103 may be considered as a hallmark of intestinal tropism. CD103 is an essential marker to identify innate and RCDII ILCs both characterized by the smCD3− CD7+ CD103+ immunophenotype. |

**Table 2** Expected distribution of lymphocytes subset in the normal gut tissue (% of lymphoid cells)

|  | Immunophenotype | IEL | LPL |
|---|---|---|---|
| TCD8+ | CD45+sm3+4−8+ | 60–80% | 40–60% |
| TCD4+ | CD45+sm3+4+8− | 5–15% | 40–60% |
| T TCRαβ+ | CD45+sm3+αβ+γδ− | 60–90% | 60–70% |
| T TCRγδ+ | CD45+sm3+αβ−γδ+ | 5–20% | 30–40% |
| ILCs | CD45+smCD3−7+103+ | 2–20% | 1–2% |
| B | CD45+smCD3−CD19+20+ | <1% | <1% |

powerful tool to dissect the lymphoid distribution in the gut tissue in high resolution (Table 2). In this regard, it is considered as the gold standard technique to ascertain the RCDII or EATL stage of the disease. Previous studies have demonstrated higher sensitivity of flow cytometry as compared to immunohistochemistry (IHC) and clonality assessment, especially if the frequency of abnormal IELs is less than 50%. IHC may miss the diagnosis of RCDII when IELs comprise 20–50% of IEL [20, 24]. This is partly explained by the capacity of flow cytometry to accurately distinguish between iCD3 and smCD3 which IHC cannot. As a result, a key IHC criterion for diagnosis is an increase in CD3+CD8− cells, but an increase in aberrant IELs can be compensated by a concomitant decrease in normal CD3+TCRγδ T-cells, which is commonly the case in RCDII [25]. This is relevant since a CD3+CD8− immunophenotype includes CD3+CD4+ and CD3+ TCRγδ T-cells. This prevents the total amount of CD3+CD8− lymphoid cells to exceed the cut-off level. It is also reported that a lack in specificity of IHC may also lead to confusion with other diseases that include an influx of CD3+CD4+ or CD3+TCRγδ+ IEL, and may erroneously classify these as RCDII. In addition, IHC presents a large interobserver variability while flow cytometry results are more robust and objective for the interpretation. The sensitivity of clonality assessment is also limited when the fraction of ILCs ranges between 20 and 50% of IELs. The exact reason for this is not clear but it may reflect the progressive transformation of normal polyclonal cells to the aberrant clonal expansion of ILCs, with a transient and intermediate oligoclonal stage. Alternatively, it may result from the low frequency of ILCs that are a minor fraction of TCR-rearranged lymphoid cells that outcompetes with other TCR-rearranged and -expressing cells in the clonality assay.

The downside of flow cytometric analysis of IELs for diagnosis of immune enteropathies is the requirement for fresh duodenal biopsies and their fast shipment to the lab, elaborate preanalytical processing as well as skilled analysts. Although flow cytometry is easily applicable and widely available it is mostly performed in reference centers. In addition, even though it represents a sensitive and reasonably specific technique to discriminate RCD and EATL from other diseases that do not associate with expansion of ILCs in IELs, it does not precisely classify the detected CeD-related lymphoma. There is no clear immunophenotype specific to EATL with exception of the above-mentioned marker combination which are suitable for orientation, but insufficient for differential diagnosis. Histopathology plays an important complementary role for the precise classification into RCDII or EATL. In other words, flow cytometry is good to detect but poor to classify CeD-related lymphoma, making this tool extremely powerful when the ILC-like RCDII IELs represent 20% to 50% of IELs, but less competitive to histomorphology and clonality assessment when this threshold is surpassed.

# Genetic Characteristics of RCDII and EATL. Application for Diagnosis

As discussed in the chapter by Cording et al., CD-associated lymphomagenesis results from the clonal expansion of unusual ILC-IELs that bear hybrid NK- and T-cell characteristics and usually show rearrangement of their TCR loci as an immunogenetic hallmark of their T-lineage affiliation. Moreover, recent data support the appearance of somatic mutations of oncogenes and anti-oncogenes that promote and sustain oncogenesis, with mutations affecting the JAK/STAT pathway among others. Molecular detection of the clonal nature of the lymphoid expansion can take advantage of both immunogenetic and oncogenetic characteristics. The following discusses the clonality assessment procedure as it is validated in the current routine diagnostic setting. The subsequent section summarizes how oncogenetic characterization can help with providing similar information, although this novel technique has not been broadly applied in the clinical work-up yet.

## *Immunogenetic Features: Clonality Assessment*

### Rationale

The T-cell receptor (TCR) is a surface antigen receptor that mediates the interaction of a T-cell with an antigenic epitope. The complementary determining region 3 (CDR3) is a particular domain of the TCR protein that closely interacts with the epitope and constitutes the proper paratope [26]. The latter represents a highly variable region for the recognition of a wide range of peptidic antigens. The tremendous diversity of antigen receptors stems from genetic recombination occurring during early stages of T-cell lymphopoiesis. Random assembly of a large set of variable (V), diversity (D), and joining (J) genes, and pairing of both chains of these heterodimeric receptors provide substantial combinatorial diversity. The latter is considerably enhanced by the so-called junctional diversity resulting from random addition and removal of some nucleotides after DNA excision and before DNA repair, generating overall $>2.5 \times 10^7$ unique TCR receptors [2, 13]. Hence, rearrangements of TCR genes constitutes a unique molecular markers for T lymphocytes. As, in most instances, tumor cells are the progeny of a single transformed malignant cell, analysis of antigen receptor gene rearrangements provides a method for clonality assessment of lymphoid proliferations [27–30]. This is usually performed by multiplexed and fluorescent PCR covering the different V(D)J segments followed by capillary electrophoresis to measure the size of the resulting PCR products. Alternatively, the PCR products may be sequenced by Sanger or next generation sequencing (NGS) to detect a dominant V(D)J recombinant and to determine its exact sequence. However, the first technique is widely used for clinical assessment, by contrast to sequencing which is usually not performed yet, as discussed below.

CeD is a dysimmune condition with no clonal expansion. Transformation to a low-grade lymphoma in RCDII and clonal expansion of iCD3+ILC-like IELs is associated with a switch to a clonal TCRγ classically detected in RCDII [31]. Similarly, EATL is associated with the detection of clonal T-cells [19, 31]. Whenever the patient is diagnosed with an RCDII and then transform into a high-grade lymphoma, the same TCRγ clone is detected in the EATL. From this arises the concept of progressive transformation of a cryptic to overt lymphoma arguing for a stepwise lymphomagenic process.

## Clonality Assessment in Clinical Practice and Technical Considerations

TCRγ genes have been a preferential target for T-lineage clonality assessment. Rearrangement of TCR loci is a physiologically sequential and ordered process with TCRδ being rearranged first, followed by TCRγ, TCRβ and finally TCRα. Therefore, any T-cell from the γδ or αβ lineage has rearranged the TCRγ locus. The TCRδ could also be considered as a relevant choice; however, the δ locus is embedded within the TCRα locus. Rearrangement of the TCRα locus results in deletion of the TCRδ locus so that it cannot be used to analyze clonality of T-cells from the αβ-lineage. In addition, the limited number of TCRγV and TCRγJ genes allows for their amplification with a small set of primers and makes the exploration of this locus easily applicable. Standardization of the molecular detection of lymphoid clonality was achieved almost 15 years ago within a European consortium involving over 45 laboratories (BIOMED-2 Concerted Action BMH4 CT98–3936, hereafter named EuroClonality) [32]. This resulted in a series of robust and highly reliable, polymerase chain reaction (PCR)-based assays, along with interpretation guidelines, which are now widely used in diagnostic laboratories [33]. The EuroClonality/

BIOMED-2 TCRγ assay was designed as a 2-tube multiplex PCR with two fluoro-chromes. No TCRγJP primer was included in order to avoid amplification of invari-ant, "canonical" TCRγ9-TCRγJP rearrangements, thus preventing their false identification as a clonal product [34]. TCRγ primers were positioned in such a way that they allowed TCRγ gene identification based on the size of the PCR products. Labeling the two reverse primers with different fluorochromes also permitted dis-tinction of TCRγJ1/2 and TCRγJP1/2 genes using GeneScan analysis. Therefore, in addition to clonality assessment, this assay could be used for partial TCRγ genotyp-ing of malignant T-cell populations. Analysis of T-cell lineage clonality is particu-larly prone to interpretation issues, as clonal rearrangements can be detected in non-malignant conditions including those associated with perturbed and restricted immune repertoires, such as chronic infection [35, 36], auto-immune disease [37–39], bone marrow transplantation [40] as well as in elderly individuals [41, 42]. Finally, disproportionate amplification of TCR gene rearrangements from rare T-cells in the sample containing only few lymphocytes can generate a seemingly clonal profile, termed pseudoclonality [33]. Although the Biomed-2 design over-comes many of these pitfalls, a drawback of this approach in the context of diagnos-tic hematopathology is that the PCR products are scattered over a wide size range and cluster according to distinct TCRγV-TCRγJ combinations. As a consequence, polyclonal T lymphocytes demonstrating rare TCRγV-TCRγJ rearrangements, for example those using TCRγV11, are at risk of being mistaken for a clonal popula-tion, due to the absence of a polyclonal background for that type of rearrangement. As a consequence, alternative approaches well-suited to the analysis of FFPE sam-ples were developed to reduce the number of false-positive results [43, 44]. The EuroClonality consortium developed an alternative TCRγ multiplex PCR assay with the particular specifications: i) to regroup PCR products within a limited size range by modifying primer positions in order to avoid over-interpretation of minor peaks of unknown significance; ii) to combine all primers within a single tube; iii) to generate relatively short PCR products (<200 bp) to facilitate analysis of FFPE samples in diagnostic pathology laboratories. Such an approach allows more robust assessment of cryopreserved and FFPE digestive tissues at diagnosis and follow-up of enteropathies with villous atrophy, thus better guiding therapeutic manage-ment [44].

TCRγ clonality by PCR characteristically demonstrates a polyclonal profile in CeD/RCDI and a clonal profile in RCDII/EATL [24, 45]. It should be noted though that clonal TCRγ products are seen in ~10% of CeD and ~20% of RCDI [46, 47]. Conversely, TCRγ rearrangement may be lacking in RCDII for various possible reasons: i) problems of interpretation as polyclonal/clonal products may be difficult to distinguish because of an intermediate or reactive dysimmune-related oligoclonal profile; ii) limitation of the informativity of the PCR, which may require analysis of the TCRδ and TCRβ loci in those cases to improve clonality detection [11, 45]; iii) competition of reactive/dysimmune T-cells hiding clonal rearrangement of rare abnormal cells within the gaussian distribution of reactive polyclonal T-cells. Another hypothesis for the lack of detected TCRγ rearrangement is related to the fact that clonal rearrangement may not be strictly synchronous with expansion of IELs which may be phenotypically detected earlier (or sometimes later on, explaining the clonal cases of CeD/RCDI). As a result, up to 25% of RCDII cases may lack clonal rearrangements of all TCR loci [17, 48]. It has been shown that up to 70% of RCDII cases with clonal TCR gene rearrangements display incomplete or out-of-frame rearrangements [20, 31]. This is consistent with the absence of smCD3 and smTCR and innate-like T IEL counterpart got blocked at an early stage of maturation.

Altogether, TCRγ clonality is widely analyzed as a first approach to differentiate RCDI from RCDII. However, clonality assessment requires a highly skilled staff and knowledge of the disease to properly differentiate polyclonal, oligoclonal and monoclonal profiles. Reproducible multicenter distinction is difficult to achieve with variability in terms of analytical sensitivity and interpretation of minor clonal populations as weak clonal rearrangements within irregular polyclonal repertoires. And even when such performance is achieved, there may be discrepancies in the disease status and the clonality profile so that TCR rearrangement data alone should not be used to diagnose RCDII. Hence, assessment of IEL clonality by TCR gene rearrangement analysis is important but not sufficient for RCDII diagnosis.

## Future Developments

Recent technical development in genetics has allowed the massive parallel sequencing of many genes or gene segments at the single-DNA molecule level. This technology usually named next-generation sequencing (NGS) has entered clinical laboratories and is now widely used to sequence oncogenes for diagnosis, prognosis stratification, theranostics and/or research. The Euroclonality group from the ESLHO foundation has been working on adapting this technique to the investigation of the TCR loci. This technology offers several advantages: i) it does not solely size PCR products but also provides the sequence of all CDR3 of single-DNA molecules; ii) it enables exploration of all rearranged T-cells and is not restricted to the dominant clone. As a result, it is expected that this technique will give new insight into the V-usage in a clinical setting and into characteristics of the CDR3 sequences. In addition, it will certainly provide information about the surrounding reactive/ residual T-cells such as TCRγδ, for which we know that their subsets according to the V-usage may have clinical significance. A recent study suggests such a value by demonstrating that TCR high-throughput-sequencing reveals a significant decrease in T-cell diversity and identifies dominant clonotypes which appear not to be gliadin-dependent in the context of RCDII [49]. In other words, resolution of immunogenetics NGS will enable precise exploration of the smoldering or dominant clone(s) and of the repertoire of polyclonal/oligoclonal T-cells to give an overview of both the clonal and polyclonal composition. In-depth understanding of the details of the clonality and of the gut immunome is a technical challenge currently under development, but it represents a promising tool in the near future to investigate the disease from both an immunological and oncological perspective.

## *Oncogenetic Features*

Although results of cytogenetic and NGS analyses are not incorporated in the current diagnostic algorithm of RCD, abnormalities detected by these assays can be useful in establishing clonality and diagnosing RCDII.

### Cytogenetics

The increase in proliferation and survival of innate IELs in RCDII makes them increasingly vulnerable to genotoxic stressors. Loss of heterozygosity at 9p21, involving the cell cycle inhibitor CDKN2A/B locus, was reported in 56% of cases and loss of 17p12-p13.2 (TP53) was detected in 23%. Aberrant nuclear p53 expression, indicative of P53 dysregulation [50], and decreased PCNA expression [48] has been observed in RCDII IELs, suggesting impaired DNA damage response and repair mechanisms. Recurrent gain of chromosome 1q22-q44 has also been detected in RCDII [11, 23], but the biological significance of this aberration is unknown. Many other abnormalities have been identified. These chromosomal abnormalities are not searched for in routine practice, but it is assumed that they contribute to the oncogenic process such as TP53 and CDKN2A. The main reason for not using cytogenetics in the diagnostic work-up is that it is difficult to get reliable information in clinical practice. The preanalytical step may be a limiting factor and IELs expansion requires being significant because of the restricted sensitivity of the technique. This may change in the near future with development of new techniques with low preanalytical constraints and high sensitivity as analysis of long range information at high coverage promises. Optical genome mapping collects up to 1500× coverage of long reads to uncover large structural variations beyond of what can be detected by short and long read sequencing, at variant allele fractions as low as 1%. Such tool is particularly well-suited to the analysis of CeD-related lymphomas and will allow for detection chromosomal abnormalities despite low infiltration in a more robust manner.

### Gene Sequencing

Rationale

Targeted next generation sequencing (TNGS) has enabled the single DNA molecule sequencing of numerous genes with a far higher sensitivity than Sanger sequencing. It enabled the genetic investigation of the disease in which tumor-cells represent a minor fraction of cells, as they are embedded in a pool of other reactive lymphoid and resident non-haematopoietic cells. TNGS provided thereby a new insight into the genetic landscape of many (pre-)malignant diseases. Recent studies have recently reported the genetic landscape of RCDII and EATL, and highlighted new concepts regarding the lymphomagenesis and maintenance of the disease [51, 52]. NGS studies are changing the understanding of the physiopathology and raised new potential druggable targets which are beyond the scope of this chapter (see Cording et al. for description of the genetic landscape and its implication in physiopathology). The clinical utility of NGS has not been deciphered yet, but as this technique is becoming broadly applicable and increasingly popular, it will certainly become an integrative part of the diagnostic work-up in the near future. The possibilities seem unlimited: TNGS may contribute to the diagnosis by demonstrating clonality, eventually subsetting the disease, or monitoring the disease during the course of treatment. Gene mutations could also be associated with a prognostic value in terms of risk of transformation into EATL, life expectancy or severity of the disease. Finally, as identification of molecular abnormalities may pave the way for discovery of druggable targets, one could also expect NGS to be able to predict sensitivity or to identify genetic determinants for drug resistance acquired during therapy as exemplified in a growing number of oncological models. This opens the avenue for possible theranostic applications. NGS is a cutting edge technique and the exact value of the tool in the care setting remains to be fully explored. In this chapter, we deal with the main pathways that have been found genetically deregulated in the context of RCDII/EATL and how it can translate into clinics. Accurate knowledge of the technique and its limitations, and of the gene mapping and functional consequences of genetic variants in the specific context of RCDII/EATL is of utmost importance to get technically reliable and clinically relevant information. This knowledge is presented here excluding conceptual and physiopathological aspects which are dealt with elsewhere (see Cording et al).

## Molecular Abnormalities in RCD and EATL

### JAK-STAT Pathway

Genes of the JAK-STAT pathway are the most commonly mutated in RCDII IELs, and they confer hyper-responsiveness to IL15 [17]. JAK1 is the top-one mutated gene with activating mutation in ~50% of RCDII, followed by STAT3 (~40%), and inactivating mutations in the negative regulators SOC1 (~15%) and SOCS3 (~10%). Overall, ~85% of RCDII patients have at least one somatic alteration of the JAK1-STAT3 axis, and multiple hits within the pathway are frequent, consisting of biallelic mutations of the same gene and/or mutations of several genes involved in the JAK1-STAT3 and its regulation. The presence of multiple hits affecting the JAK1-STAT3 pathway favors a synergistic role of combined mutations, which is further supported by the demonstration that concomitant STAT3 and JAK1 mutations can cooperatively amplify STAT3 activation [53]. This is also consistent with other disease model in which JAK-STAT pathway plays a driver role with a significant frequency and in which up to 30% of multiple hits can be seen [54].

Topographic mapping of the recurrent JAK1 mutations show that they cluster in ~95% of cases at the p.G1097 position in the C-terminal JH1-kinase domain, a highly conserved position, and the site of interaction with the JAK1 negative regulator SOCS1 [55]. Within this hotspot, the p.G1097D variant is most frequent (~58%), followed by p.G1097V/C/S/R (~25%, ~8%, ~4% and ~4%, respectively) [51]. Of note, almost all JAK1 not located in the JAK1 p.G1097 hotspot co-occur with a JAK1 p.G1097 hotspot mutation. STAT3 mutations cluster in the STAT3 SH2 domain with a tiny minority of mutations in the coiled-coil or DNA binding domains. Alike JAK1, virtually all STAT3 mutations not located in the STAT3 SH2 domain co-occur with a JAK1 p.G1097 hotspot mutation. SOCS1 and SOCS3 mutations do not show specific hotspot localization consistent with their lower frequency and their loss-of-function (LOF) impact. All functionally tested cases show constitutive and/or enhanced cytokine-driven phosphorylation of STAT3. Some cases without documented mutation of the pathway may still show increased phosphorylation of STAT3. This raises the technical issue of possible genetic alterations not captured by the sequencing strategy but also the potential biological consequence of epigenetic changes without a genetic hit affecting the JAK-STAT pathway itself.

Mutations of the JAK-STAT pathway play a driver role in RCDII by inducing constitutive or hypersensitive cytokine-driven phosphorylation of STAT3. This pattern is pretty unique to RCDII/EATL but has also been reported in some ALK-negative anaplastic lymphomas (8%) including those developing on breast implants (18%) [53, 56]. Its frequency is however less than in RCDII and EATL (50% and 68%, respectively), suggesting that JAK1 p.G1097 mutations are a hallmark of RCDII and may be a diagnostic marker for CeD-related lymphomas given its relative specificity [57].

### Other Genes Mutations

A constellation of other genes may be found mutated, some of which are recurrently affected. Mutations of the NF-κB regulating genes are recurrent (~22%) in RCDII and affect the negative regulators TNFAIP3 (13%) and TNIP3 (9%) [51, 52]. They are mostly missense, nonsense or frameshift mutations indicating their deleterious nature. Other frequent mutations affect epigenetic modifiers TET2 (~30%) and KMT2D (~25%). Both mutations are almost all predicted loss-of-function mutations consisting of nonsense and frameshift mutations that result in truncated and nonfunctional proteins. TET2 mutations are seen in numerous hematological malignancies of myeloid origin (acute myeloid leukemia, myeloproliferative neoplasms, myelodysplasia, clonal haematopoiesis), but are also well-known in context of mature T-cell lymphoid malignancies in particular in particular in angioimmunoblastic T-cell lymphoma (AITL) [58]. In the context of gut diseases, TET2 mutations are also observed in EATL and MEITL. Somatic variants of DDX3X (~20%), an RNA helicase, may be found with constant loss-of-function mutations consisting of mainly truncating frameshift or missense mutations. Genes involved in DNA damage response and repair may be affected. POT1 is a telomere-binding protein that protects the broken chromosome ends from fusion and degradation that may be mutated, but again with a low specificity as it is genetically altered in other subtypes of T-cell lymphomas. Related genes such as CCND3 and CHEK1 are occasionally mutated. CD58 is an immune evasion molecules that interacts with CD2 expressed on T/NK cells to prevent immune recognition and fratricidie. Inactivating mutations of CD58 are found in RCDII and likewise in other subtypes of T-cell lymphoma such as Adult T-cell Lymphoma/Leukemia (ATLL) [59].

*Lessons from the VAFs*

While Sanger sequencing provides dichotomic information regarding the presence or absence of somatic mutations, NGS enables semi-quantitative determination of the somatic variant load. This represents interesting information about the tumor load and allows comparison of relative somatic variant frequencies from which the clonal structure can be inferred. This is reflected in the variant allelic frequency (VAF), a parameter that consists of the ratio of the number of alternative reads divided by the total number of reads ($Reads^{Alt}/(Reads^{Alt} + Reads^{WT})$). Recent studies have not deciphered the clonal structure and its evolution in RCDII yet. However, frequently high VAF of JAK1 and STAT3 mutations probably reflect biallelic mutations. From a practical perspective, it increases the likelihood to pick-up the variant in low-infiltrated samples. From a biological view, it strengthens again the oncogenic effect of the JAK1-STAT3 activation that is achieved by multiple hits within the pathway (multigenic event), within the same gene (heterozygote composites), or at the same location (homozygocytic mutation). High VAF also supports the driver role of the pathway in lymphomagenesis although it has not been formally demonstrated yet whether JAK1-STAT3 mutations act as drivers or founders. As an alternative mechanism, loss-of-heterozygosity may be induced by focal or large deletion, or by uniparental disomy (UPD). However, these phenomenons are difficult to reveal with routine diagnostic tools given the often low infiltration rate of the tissue. High VAF can also be seen in TET2, as well as heterozygous composite. DDX3X also show high VAF in men, which is related to the location on X chromosome of this gene.

Overall, the studies show relatively low VAF as compared to other lymphoid malignancies, ranging from ~1 to 30%. This suggests that some mutations may be unseen in low-infiltrated samples, and/or when abnormalities are subclonal. The latter situation is plausible as suggested by the variability of the VAFs within individual samples supporting intratumour heterogeneity. Of note, some associations can be observed as it seems that STAT3 mutations significantly co-occur with TET2 mutations while JAK1 mutations tend to be mutually exclusive with STAT3 and TET2. The biological relevance of this observation remains unclear, but it may reflect a stronger oncogenic effect of JAK1 alone while STAT3 may require to synergize with TET2. Knowledge of these associations may facilitate the interpretation of the NGS analysis in practice.

Clinical Significance

Acquisition by a subset of IELs of somatic GOF mutations in the JAK-STAT pathway represents a decisive step in the progression towards s lymphomas complicating CeD. It translates into the clinic by the fact that the JAK1/STAT3 and other above-mentioned somatic mutations segregate with the previously defined entities. Somatic mutations are inexistent in CeD and RCDI. By contrast, at least one mutation affecting the JAK1/STAT3 axis is found in 78% of RCDII and 93% of EATL. This provides a strong evidence for clonality and progression to the lymphomatous stage. While immunogenetic analysis of the TCRγ locus contributes to the diagnosis with evidence of clonal expansion, it is not specific to the underlying disease. Somatic mutations help with the differential diagnosis with some mutations evoking a more specific lymphoma. For instance, identification in the duodenum tissue of a *JAK1* G1097D mutation (*a fortiori* if it is homozygous), or a combination of STAT3 GOF and TET2 LOF mutations in the context of CeD with recurrence of histopathological signs is a strong indicator of evolution to the lymphoma stage of the disease (RCDII or EATL). By contrast, identification of a combination of SETD2 LOF and TET2 LOF with no context of CeD will favor a diagnosis of MEITL, as SETD2 mutations have rarely been detected in RCDII or EATL. Still, the exact value of NGS in the diagnostic work-up remains to be determined and it will complement it rather than replacing other existing tests. The sensitivity of NGS assays is a critical limitation as it is highly dependent on the tumor load of malignant cells. It is likely that somatic mutations are rather undetected but not necessarily absent from the tissue sample in cases without reported mutations. This limitation results from the competition of the unmutated DNA molecules from all nucleated cells present in the sample. This limitation is not the same with TCRγ clonality analysis which can pick up a clonal TCRγ rearrangement present in only a few T-IELs among thousands of epithelial cells. The limitation of TCRγ clonality is restricted to the presence and competition with other polyclonal T-cells. Because the technique relies on sizing rather than sequencing, it results in a gaussian curve for polyclonal T-cells from which clonal rearrangements- emerge as peaks (Fig. 2). As a consequence, the more polyclonal T-cells are present, the less sensitive the assay, and the more the size of the rearrangement deviates from the median, the more sensitive the assay. By contrast, all other surrounding nucleated cells have no impact on the sensitivity of the clonality assay as their TCR loci remain in a germinal state. Whenever a clonal expansion doesn't show any TCRγ rearrangement, it may also be related to competition of reactive T-cells or the hybrid T/NK origin and immaturity of innate-like IELs that may lack TCRγ rearrangements. The relative sensitivity of the immunogenetic and oncogenetic clonality assays is not clear yet, but it is likely that NGS will provide complementary rather than substituting information as the biological determinants for the sensitivity differ between the techniques.

As TCRγ clonality analysis, NGS is able to identify the evolution into a lymphoma stage. However, there is no genetic pattern specific to the cryptic or the overt lymphoma entities. In line with this, no mutation predicts the evolution into EATL

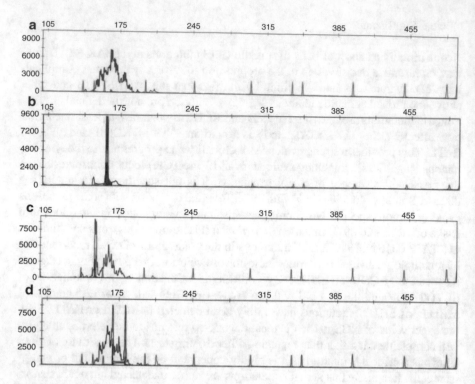

**Fig. 2** Representative examples of molecular assessment of clonality using the BIOMED-2 tube in duodenal biopsies of different patients. Green line, Vγ-JP1 rearrangements; blue line, Vγ-Jγ rearrangements; red line, ladder; X-axis, size of the rearrangements, Y-axis, fluorescence intensity. (**a**) Polyclonal TCRγ profile, (**b**) clonal TCRγ profile, (**c**) clonal TCRγ profile with a polyclonal TCRγ background, (**d**) two clonal rearrangements, one clearly visible because of extreme size, the other less clear because of a medium size embedded in the Gaussian curve of polyclonal background generated by normal residual T-cells

yet, nor does the number of mutations. Moreover, no genetic pattern with a prognostic impact has been identified so far. Currently, there is no available biomarker to predict evolution into EATL, and histopathology is the only diagnostic tool to discriminate between RCDII and EATL at the time of transformation. EATL is a rare disease and the genetic landscape has only been investigated in limited series. A collaborative effort will be required to extend the size of the cohorts and to create confirmatory/validation cohorts. This could allow for the identification of genetic markers to predict the evolution of RCDII into EATL or identify genetic alterations pathognomonic of EATL. To date, longitudinal and pairwise analyses of sequential samples from RCDII to EATL did not reveal accumulation of recurrent genetic hits. Likewise, another issue that remains unresolved is the question of whether the genetic content may differ between de novo and post-RCDII EATLs. No difference has been highlighted in previous series but again, this might be due to the limited numbers of patients involved in these studies.

Technical Aspects

NGS allows for the investigation of many genes in a single assay with high resolution (~1%). To achieve such sensitivity, NGS involves some technical requirements. Indeed, background noise and sequencing errors represent a significant fraction of reads (~1%), which often overlap with the underlying somatic mutation frequency. This holds even more true for results obtained from formalin-fixed and paraffin-embedded (FFPE) tissues, which underwent a deamidation process that impairs correct sequencing, thus adding an additional layer of noise to the intrinsic replication error of the polymerase. To circumvent such technical events that can lead to erroneous identification of mutations, some considerations must be taken into account: a) fresh or frozen samples should be preferred over FFPE samples; b) FFPE samples should be treated adequately at the pre-analytic step to reverse deamidation; c) target enrichment should preferably be achieved by the use of capture beads rather than PCR-based amplification in order to avoid the artefactual base replacement during library preparation due to the error rate of the polymerase; d) the sequencing depth should be sufficient (>300×–500×) in order to achieve optimal sensitivity; e) data curation should be performed by skilled experts with good knowledge of the expected genetic patterns and hotspots; f) whenever possible, analysis of samples prepared for immunophenotypic analysis is preferred, as separation of IELs and LPLs results in high enrichment of the target cells in the IEL fraction. In addition, while flow cytometry is quite straightforward and TCRγ clonality has benefited from strong standardization through the concerted Biomed-2 actions, NGS remains a novel technique in clinical diagnostics. Strong technical efforts for quality checks, standardization or harmonization of the analysis and quality assessment are required to obtain robust and comparable results across centers and to avoid false-positive/false-negative results in the clinical setting.

# Conclusion and Perspectives

Diagnosis of RCDII and EATL relies on a multidisciplinary approach involving histomorphology, immunochemistry, flow cytometry, and molecular biology [60, 61]. Although the diagnosis is not codified through a score, complementary diagnostic criteria of each technique are well established and diagnosis results from the confrontation of the pieces of data to build a body of evidence. HLA-typing, seric antibody detection and histomorphology are essential for the diagnosis of CeD. Flow cytometry plays a frontline role to detect CeD-induced lymphoma owing to its high sensitivity [62]. Although widely available, flow cytometry is not that often applied in many centers. It requires heavy preanalytical steps and trained experts to perform this assay reliably. Histomorphology associated with immunohistochemistry and clonality assessment are then more widely applied with a lower sensitivity though. But histomorphology and immunochemistry have to be performed in any case to type the CeD-related lymphoma as neither flow cytometry nor molecular biology are able to perform such a typing and thus remain the gold standard for differential diagnosis. Recent advances in molecular biology have been made with the advent of NGS, which nowadays reaches the clinical labs and is becoming increasingly popular. The clinical significance of this new tool remains to be established, but it offers novel insight into the disease mechanisms and is of promising value for the near future. Detection of JAK1, STAT3 and TNFAIP3 mutations are already employed as a hallmark of the disease and represent markers for clonality in some labs. It is expected that additional insight will be achieved with on-going technical developments in molecular biology. High-sensitive detection of structural chromosomal abnormalities will complete the genetic picture of the disease. From this and a better understanding of the physiopathology, one can expect an improved characterization and sub classification of the disease with regard to drug sensitivity and personalized therapeutic approaches. While clinical tools mostly contribute to the diagnostics, little is known about their utility during follow-up. Future developments should clarify how to determine the prognosis, the risk of evolution into a secondary EATL, predict sensitivity to drugs, assess the quality of the response by defining complete and partial response criteria and to detect markers of secondary resistance to targeted therapy as achieved in many oncological models of solid tumors or hematological malignancies.

# References

1. Kagnoff MF. Celiac disease: pathogenesis of a model immunogenetic disease. J Clin Invest. 2007;117(1):41–9.
2. West J. Celiac disease and its complications: a time traveller's perspective. Gastroenterology. 2009;136(1):32–4.
3. Ludvigsson JF, Leffler DA, Bai JC, et al. The Oslo definitions for coeliac disease and related terms. Gut. 2013;62(1):43–52.
4. Penny HA, Baggus EMR, Rej A, Snowden JA, Sanders DS. Non-Responsive Coeliac Disease: A Comprehensive Review from the NHS England National Centre for Refractory Coeliac Disease. Nutrients. 2020;12(1):E216.
5. Malamut G, Meresse B, Cellier C, Cerf-Bensussan N. Refractory celiac disease: from bench to bedside. Semin Immunopathol. 2012;34(4):601–13.
6. Daum S, Cellier C, Mulder CJJ. Refractory coeliac disease. Best Pract Res Clin Gastroenterol. 2005;19(3):413–24.
7. Al-toma A, Verbeek WHM, Hadithi M, von Blomberg BME, Mulder CJJ. Survival in refractory coeliac disease and enteropathy-associated T-cell lymphoma: retrospective evaluation of single-centre experience. Gut. 2007;56(10):1373–8.
8. Bagdi E, Diss TC, Munson P, Isaacson PG. Mucosal intra-epithelial lymphocytes in enteropathy-associated T-cell lymphoma, ulcerative Jejunitis, and refractory celiac disease constitute a neoplastic population. Blood. 1999;94(1):260–4.
9. Carbonnel F, Grollet-Bioul L, Brouet JC, et al. Are complicated forms of celiac disease cryptic T-cell lymphomas? Blood. 1998;92(10):3879–86.
10. Malamut G, Cellier C. Complications of coeliac disease. Best Pract Res Clin Gastroenterol. 2015;29(3):451–8.
11. Malamut G, Afchain P, Verkarre V, et al. Presentation and long-term follow-up of refractory celiac disease: comparison of type I with type II. Gastroenterology. 2009;136(1):81–90.

12. Verbeek WHM, Schreurs MWJ, Visser OJ, et al. Novel approaches in the management of refractory celiac disease. Expert Rev Clin Immunol. 2008;4(2):205–19.

13. Meresse B, Malamut G, Cerf-Bensussan N. Celiac disease: an immunological jigsaw. Immunity. 2012;36(6):907–19.

14. Nijeboer P, Malamut G, Mulder CJ, et al. Enteropathy-associated T-cell lymphoma: improving treatment strategies. Dig Dis. 2015;33(2):231–5.

15. Guy-Grand D, Cerf-Bensussan N, Malissen B, et al. Two gut intraepithelial CD8+ lymphocyte populations with different T cell receptors: a role for the gut epithelium in T cell differentiation. J Exp Med. 1991;173(2):471–81.

16. Jarry A, Cerf-Bensussan N, Brousse N, Selz F, Guy-Grand D. Subsets of CD3+ (T cell receptor alpha/beta or gamma/delta) and CD3- lymphocytes isolated from normal human gut epithelium display phenotypical features different from their counterparts in peripheral blood. Eur J Immunol. 1990;20(5):1097–103.

17. Ettersperger J, Montcuquet N, Malamut G, et al. Interleukin-15-dependent T-cell-like innate intraepithelial lymphocytes develop in the intestine and transform into lymphomas in celiac disease. Immunity. 2016;45(3):610–25.

18. Schmitz F, Tjon JML, Lai Y, et al. Identification of a potential physiological precursor of aberrant cells in refractory coeliac disease type II. Gut. 2013;62(4):509–19.

19. Cellier C, Delabesse E, Helmer C, et al. Refractory sprue, coeliac disease, and enteropathy-associated T-cell lymphoma. Lancet. 2000;356(9225):203–8.

20. Verbeek WHM, Goerres MS, von Blomberg BME, et al. Flow cytometric determination of aberrant intra-epithelial lymphocytes predicts T-cell lymphoma development more accurately than T-cell clonality analysis in refractory celiac disease. Clin Immunol. 2008;126(1):48–56.

21. Hüe S, Mention J-J, Monteiro RC, et al. A direct role for NKG2D/MICA interaction in villous atrophy during celiac disease. Immunity. 2004;21(3):367–77.

22. Verbeek WHM, von Blomberg BME, Coupe VMH, et al. Aberrant T-lymphocytes in refractory coeliac disease are not strictly confined to a small intestinal intraepithelial localization. Cytometry B Clin Cytom. 2009;76(6):367–74.

23. Verkarre V. Refractory coeliac sprue is a diffuse gastrointestinal disease. Gut. 2003;52(2):205–11.

24. van Wanrooij RLJ, Müller DMJ, Neefjes-Borst EA, et al. Optimal strategies to identify aberrant intra-epithelial lymphocytes in refractory coeliac disease. J Clin Immunol. 2014;34(7):828–35.

25. Verbeek WHM, von Blomberg BME, Scholten PET, et al. The presence of small intestinal intraepithelial gamma/delta T-lymphocytes is inversely correlated with lymphoma development in refractory celiac disease. Am J Gastroenterol. 2008;103(12):3152–8.

26. Davis MM. The evolutionary and structural 'logic' of antigen receptor diversity. Semin Immunol. 2004;16(4):239–43.

27. Akram S, Murray JA, Pardi DS, et al. Adult autoimmune enteropathy: Mayo Clinic Rochester experience. Clin Gastroenterol Hepatol. 2007;5(11):1282–45.

28. Carbonnel F, d'Almagne H, Lavergne A, et al. The clinicopathological features of extensive small intestinal CD4 T cell infiltration. Gut. 1999;45(5):662–7.

29. Cellier C, Patey N, Mauvieux L, et al. Abnormal intestinal intraepithelial lymphocytes in refractory sprue. Gastroenterology. 1998;114(3):471–81.

30. Perry AM, Warnke RA, Hu Q, et al. Indolent T-cell lymphoproliferative disease of the gastrointestinal tract. Blood. 2013;122(22):3599–606.

31. Daum S. Frequency of clonal intraepithelial T lymphocyte proliferations in enteropathy-type intestinal T cell lymphoma, coeliac disease, and refractory sprue. Gut. 2001;49(6):804–12.

32. van Dongen JJM, Langerak AW, Brüggemann M, et al. Design and standardization of PCR primers and protocols for detection of clonal immunoglobulin and T-cell receptor gene recombinations in suspect lymphoproliferations: report of the BIOMED-2 concerted action BMH4-CT98-3936. Leukemia. 2003;17(12):2257–317.

33. Langerak AW, Groenen PJTA, Brüggemann M, et al. EuroClonality/BIOMED-2 guidelines for interpretation and reporting of Ig/TCR clonality testing in suspected lymphoproliferations. Leukemia. 2012;26(10):2159–71.

34. Delfau MH, Hance AJ, Lecossier D, Vilmer E, Grandchamp B. Restricted diversity of V gamma 9-JP rearrangements in unstimulated human gamma/delta T lymphocytes. Eur J Immunol. 1992;22(9):2437–43.

35. Gamadia LE, van Leeuwen EMM, Remmerswaal EBM, et al. The size and phenotype of virus-specific T cell populations is determined by repetitive antigenic stimulation and environmental cytokines. J Immunol. 2004;172(10):6107–14.

36. Khan N, Shariff N, Cobbold M, et al. Cytomegalovirus seropositivity drives the CD8 T cell repertoire toward greater clonality in healthy elderly individuals. J Immunol. 2002;169(4):1984–92.

37. Bristeau-Leprince A, Mateo V, Lim A, et al. Human TCR alpha/beta+ CD4-CD8- double-negative T cells in patients with autoimmune lymphoproliferative syndrome express restricted Vbeta TCR diversity and are clonally related to CD8+ T cells. J Immunol. 2008;181(1):440–8.

38. Martin A, Barbesino G, Davies TF. T-cell receptors and autoimmune thyroid disease--signposts for T-cell-antigen driven diseases. Int Rev Immunol. 1999;18(1–2):111–40.

39. Ramesh M, Hamm D, Simchoni N, Cunningham-Rundles C. Clonal and constricted T cell repertoire in common variable immune deficiency. Clin Immunol. 2017;178:1–9.

40. Yew PY, Alachkar H, Yamaguchi R, et al. Quantitative characterization of T-cell repertoire in allogeneic hematopoietic stem cell transplant recipients. Bone Marrow Transplant. 2015;50(9):1227–34.

41. Lazuardi L, Jenewein B, Wolf AM, et al. Age-related loss of naïve T cells and dysregulation of T-cell/B-cell interactions in human lymph nodes. Immunology. 2005;114(1):37–43.

42. Naylor K, Li G, Vallejo AN, et al. The influence of age on T cell generation and TCR diversity. J Immunol. 2005;174(11):7446–52.

43. Armand M, Derrieux C, Beldjord K, et al. A new and simple TRG multiplex PCR assay for assessment of T-cell clonality: a comparative study from the EuroClonality consortium. Hema. 2019;3(3):e255.

44. Derrieux C, Trinquand A, Bruneau J, et al. A single-tube, EuroClonality-inspired, TRG clonality multiplex PCR aids management of patients with enteropathic diseases, including from formaldehyde-fixed, paraffin-embedded tissues. J Mol Diagn. 2019;21(1):111–22.

45. Perfetti V, Brunetti L, Biagi F, et al. TCRβ clonality improves diagnostic yield of TCRγ clonality in refractory celiac disease. J Clin Gastroenterol. 2012;46(8):675–9.

46. Hussein S, Gindin T, Lagana SM, et al. Clonal T cell receptor gene rearrangements in coeliac disease: implications for diagnosing refractory coeliac disease. J Clin Pathol. 2018;71(9):825–31.

47. Liu H, Brais R, Lavergne-Slove A, et al. Continual monitoring of intraepithelial lymphocyte immunophenotype and clonality is more important than snapshot analysis in the surveillance of refractory coeliac disease. Gut. 2010;59(4):452–60.

48. Tack GJ, van Wanrooij RLJ, Langerak AW, et al. Origin and immunophenotype of aberrant IEL in RCDII patients. Mol Immunol. 2012;50(4):262–70.

49. Ritter J, Zimmermann K, Jöhrens K, et al. T-cell repertoires in refractory coeliac disease. Gut. 2018;67(4):644–53.

50. Obermann EC, Diss TC, Hamoudi RA, et al. Loss of heterozygosity at chromosome 9p21 is a frequent finding in enteropathy-type T-cell lymphoma. J Pathol. 2004;202(2):252–62.

51. Cording S, Lhermitte L, Malamut G, et al. Oncogenetic landscape of lymphomagenesis in coeliac disease. Gut. 2021.

52. Soderquist CR, Lewis SK, Gru AA, et al. Immunophenotypic spectrum and genomic landscape of refractory celiac disease type II. Am J Surg Pathol. 2021;45(7):905–16.

53. Crescenzo R, Abate F, Lasorsa E, et al. Convergent mutations and kinase fusions lead to oncogenic STAT3 activation in anaplastic large cell lymphoma. Cancer Cell. 2015;27(4):516–32.

54. Kim R, Boissel N, Touzart A, et al. Adult T-cell acute lymphoblastic leukemias with IL7R pathway mutations are slow-responders who do not benefit from allogeneic stem-cell transplantation. Leukemia. 2020;34(7):1730–40.

55. Liau NPD, Laktyushin A, Lucet IS, et al. The molecular basis of JAK/STAT inhibition by SOCS1. Nat Commun. 2018;9(1):1558.
56. Laurent C, Nicolae A, Laurent C, et al. Gene alterations in epigenetic modifiers and JAK-STAT signaling are frequent in breast implant-associated ALCL. Blood. 2020;135(5):360–70.
57. Nicolae A, Xi L, Pham TH, et al. Mutations in the JAK/STAT and RAS signaling pathways are common in intestinal T-cell lymphomas. Leukemia. 2016;30(11):2245–7.
58. Odejide O, Weigert O, Lane AA, et al. A targeted mutational landscape of angioimmunoblastic T-cell lymphoma. Blood. 2014;123(9):1293–6.
59. Marçais A, Lhermitte L, Artesi M, et al. Targeted deep sequencing reveals clonal and subclonal mutational signatures in Adult T-cell leukemia/lymphoma and defines an unfavorable indolent subtype. Leukemia. 2021;35(3):764–76.
60. Rubio-Tapia A, Murray JA. Classification and management of refractory coeliac disease. Gut. 2010;59(4):547–57.
61. Rubio-Tapia A, Murray JA. Updated guidelines by the European Society for the Study of coeliac disease. United European Gastroenterol J. 2019;7(5):581–2.
62. van Wanrooij RLJ, Schreurs MWJ, Bouma G, et al. Accurate classification of RCD requires flow cytometry. Gut. 2010;59(12):1732.

# The Other Causes of Severe Enteropathy with Villous Atrophy Non-Responsive to a Gluten-Free Diet

Isabel A. Hujoel and Joseph A. Murray

## Environmental Enteropathy

Environmental enteropathy, sometimes referred to as tropical enteropathy, is a highly prevalent condition among poor children in low and middle-income countries, and is estimated to impact roughly 170 million children worldwide. Described as a subclinical condition, environmental enteropathy is thought to lead to the stunted growth of 1/3 of the children in these countries [1]. Although these children are seen as "asymptomatic" as they have no diarrhea, the long-term impact of environmental enteropathy is devastating as it can lead to growth impairment, decreased cognitive ability, future obesity, and poor response to oral vaccines [2]. Severe acute malnutrition is a subgroup of environmental enteropathy defined by wasting, and affects an estimated 20 million children every year [1]. The pathophysiology of environmental enteropathy and severe acute malnutrition is not yet fully understood. The leading hypothesis is that it is secondary to poor sanitation, and more specifically to chronic fecal-oral contamination. A T-cell mediated response to environmental antigen(s), such as the contents of feces, has been suggested. Studies have found high levels of and several types of pathogens in children in low-income countries [3]. While these pathogens may not cause diarrhea, it is thought that their presence leads to epithelial damage, increased intestinal permeability, and impaired gut immune function. One recent study examining children with severe acute malnutrition found that they had evidence of bacterial translocation and increased intestinal permeability [1]. The intestinal damage is believed to explain the failure of children to respond to nutritional interventions, and the inefficacy of oral vaccines [4–6]. Pathology shows findings similar to celiac disease with villous blunting, crypt hyperplasia, and lymphocytic infiltration of lamina propria [7]. At this point,

I. A. Hujoel · J. A. Murray (✉)
Division of Gastroenterology and Hepatology, Mayo Clinic, Rochester, MN, USA
e-mail: isabelh@uw.edu; murray.joseph@mayo.edu

© Springer Nature Switzerland AG 2022
G. Malamut, N. Cerf-Bensussan (eds.), *Refractory Celiac Disease*,
https://doi.org/10.1007/978-3-030-90142-4_8

although there have been studies on medications such as rifaximin and mesalamine, these do not appear to be effective, and no clear therapy is available.

## Autoimmune Enteropathy

Autoimmune enteropathy (AIE) is a rare condition, with an incidence of 1/100,000. The disease most commonly affects infants but is being increasingly seen in adults who are typically middle-aged and often have a co-existent autoimmune disease [8, 9]. Cases associated with thymomas have also been reported [10]. In children, AIE is commonly related to an underlying genetic mutation, while in adults it is instead thought to be a collection of different conditions that share underlying dysregulation of the immune system [11].

Two pediatric systemic forms of AIE include immune dysregulation, polyendocrinopathy, enteropathy, X-linked (IPEX) syndrome, and autoimmune polyendocrinopathy, candidiasis, and ectodermal dystrophy (APECED) syndrome [12]. These are related to loss of function mutations in FOXP3 and an autoimmune regulatory gene respectively. More rare variants of AIE include monogenic disorders that impact T-regulatory cells (such as mutations in the interleukin 2 receptor α chain (IL2Ra) gene and a missense mutation in the mucosa-associated lymphoid tissue lymphoma translocation 1 gene (MALT1)) and T effector cells (such as gain of function mutations in STAT3 and mutations in cytotoxic T-lymphocyte 4 protein precursor (CTLA-4) or LPS-responsive beige-like anchor (LRBA)) [13, 14].

AIE presents with severe malabsorption. Children present with severe diarrhea, weight loss, and failure to thrive. With IPEX there is often coexistent endocrinopathies and insulin dependent diabetes. These children mostly die prior to the age of 3 unless treated with a hematopoietic stem cell transplant. Children with APECED can also present with adrenal gland insufficiency and hypoparathyroidism, and can survive until adolescence. Adults most commonly present with severe weight loss, chronic diarrhea, and malabsorption [8, 9].

Diagnosis of AIE relies on the Mayo Clinic criteria which include: 1) chronic diarrhea over 6 weeks in duration 2) malabsorption, 3) specific small bowel histology (partial or complete villous blunting with minimal intraepithelial lymphocytosis), and 4) exclusion of other causes of villous atrophy [8]. Symptoms and histologic damage need to have no response to dietary exclusions, including gluten. While classically immunodeficiency needs to be excluded in order to make a diagnosis of AIE, there have been studies linking immunodeficiency with AIE. One study identified a deficiency in NFAT5, which regulates inflammation and the immune response, in a patient with AIE and primary immunodeficiency syndrome [15]. Testing three other AIE patients identified heterozygous variants, suggesting uniparental disomy in all. Anti-enterocyte and goblet cells are suggestive of AIE but are not required for diagnosis and do not play a pathogenic role in disease development. The antibodies are not specific and can be seen in other diseases. Endoscopy typically shows nonspecific changes. Histopathologic findings are variable, but roughly 20% of cases will present with celiac-like changes including villous atrophy and crypt abscess. Often there is no significant intraepithelial lymphocytosis [9]. Paneth or Goblet cells may be absent.

AIE can be difficult to treat, with only 50% having complete response and up to 50% needing total parenteral nutrition. Initially topically active steroids are used, such as budesonide (3 mg three times daily) adapted to deliver to the affected parts of the intestine. If this fails, then treatment can escalate to a systemic steroid such as prednisone at a dose of 30 to 60 mg daily. Methylprednisolone (40–50 mg IV daily) can also be used initially in very ill adults. Steroid sparing agents include azathioprine, 6-mercaptopurine, cyclosporine, tacrolimus and infliximab. Case reports describe the use of ustekinumab and vedolizumab [16]. Hematopoietic stem cell transplant can be considered in children with IPEX, and there have been case reports of targeted therapy based on the underlying mutation (for example the use of the JAK ½ inhibitor ruxolitinib in a child with a STAT3 gain of function mutation) [13].

## Common Variable Immunodeficiency Enteropathy

Common variable immunodeficiency has a prevalence of 1/250,000 to 1/10,000 and typically is diagnosed in the mid-30s. Digestive symptoms lead to diagnosis in up to 40% of cases, and up to 50% of cases suffer from chronic diarrhea and malabsorption [17]. These symptoms are often related to infections, which in order of decreasing frequency include *Giardia lamblia* (Herman's syndrome), *Campylobacter jejuni*, and *Salmonella* [17]. They can also be secondary to enteropathies that resemble either inflammatory bowel disease or celiac disease.

Most cases of CVID are sporadic, however 20% are familial. CVID is secondary to mutations that affect B-cell function and differentiation. A mutation in the trans membrane activator and calcium-modulating cyclophilin ligand interactor (TACI) is present in up to 10% of cases [18]. It is not known why individuals with CVID develop enteropathy, however there are hypotheses that involve the absence of intestinal plasma cells and a defect in secretory antibodies leading to chronic infections which in turn leads to chronic inflammation. Both a deficiency in secretory IgA is postulated causing anaerobic bacterial overgrowth and an abnormal CD4+/CD8+ ratio have also been implicated.

Symptoms in order of decreasing frequency include diarrhea, dyspepsia, and abdominal pain. Diminished response to vaccines and recurrent infections may also be seen. Diagnosis requires two of the three major immunoglobulin classes (IgA, IgG, IgM) to be two standard deviations below normal. Additionally, there should be an impaired antibody response to vaccinations or infections, and other causes of immunodeficiency need to be excluded. Laboratory studies may show malnutrition and anemia and auto-antibodies and peripheral lymphocytic abnormalities can be seen [17]. Evaluation of chronic diarrhea in the setting of CVID should include both upper endoscopy and colonoscopy with biopsies. Abnormalities on endoscopic examination are common and in the small intestine there may be nodular lymphoid hyperplasia (44%), loss of folds (22%), and ulcerative duodenitis (2%). Histology from the small intestine is notable for absence of plasma cells in 83% of cases. Polymorphonuclear infiltrates and apoptotic cells may also be seen. Roughly three quarters of individuals will have increased intraepithelial lymphocytes, which in half is associated with villous atrophy. Findings can extend into the colon, where the most common finding is microscopic colitis [16].

A celiac-like presentation is common in those with CVID, and identifying the presence of true celiac disease can be difficult, as serologic results are often misleading, and CVID enteropathy related symptoms and villous atrophy may respond to a gluten-free diet [17, 19]. HLA typing can be helpful in identifying those who are genetically susceptible to celiac disease, and lack of response to a gluten-free diet can exclude those with celiac disease. One study found that those without permissive haplotypes were more likely to have an expansion of B cells with low CD21 expression [20].

Intravenous immunoglobulin is the treatment for CVID. Although it reduces infection rate, it is not generally effective in reducing gastrointestinal symptoms. Frequently, individuals with CVID-associated enteropathy will need parenteral nutrition. Any co-existent infections, especially SIBO, should be treated, and oral steroids (such as prednisone at a dose of 10 mg per day or budesonide 3 mg three times daily) can have significant beneficial impact. Infliximab and etanercept have also been used in those with CVID with granuloma formation with some success [21].

# Lymphoproliferative Disorders

The gastrointestinal tract, due to its constant exposure to foreign antigens, has a significant amount of lymphoid tissue. Perhaps related to this, it has numerous potential lymphoproliferative disorders, and is the most common extranodal site for lymphomas, most of which are B-cell [22, 23]. The most common lymphoproliferative disorders that can present with villous atrophy include type 1 enteropathy-associated T-cell lymphoma (EATL), type 2 EATL, indolent T-cell lymphoproliferative disorders, and mucosa-associated lymphoid tissue (MALT) lymphoma.

Type 1 and type 2 EATL vary significantly in their associations and demographics. Type 1 is more prevalent (80–90%) than type 2 (10–20%). Type 1 EATL is associated with celiac disease, and as a consequence of this is seen predominantly in populations with a higher prevalence of celiac disease, such as Northern Europeans. Although it makes up only 5% of peripheral T-cell lymphomas, it is the most common primary intestinal lymphoma in the West. It commonly is preceded by refractory celiac disease, although not always, and generally occurs around mid-life (50s) and slightly more often in men. Typically, individuals present with abdominal pain, diarrhea, and weight loss. They may also present with perforation and obstruction. Endoscopically, ulceration may be seen as well as strictures. On histology, an inflammatory infiltrate and villous blunting as well as a mass lesion with an extensive lymphoid infiltration can be seen. EATL has a very poor prognosis and can be treated with chemotherapy and in some cases an autologous stem cell transplant.

Type 2 EATL, also called monomorphic epitheliotropic intestinal T-cell lymphoma (MEITL) by contrast, is not associated with celiac disease as frequently and is more common in Asian populations. It is more prevalent in males and also generally occurs in the fifth decade of life. Presentation can range from diarrhea and weight loss to bowel perforation in over half of the cases. The jejunum tends to be involved, but the disease can spread through the entire gastrointestinal tract. One or more tumors may be present and ulceration may be seen endoscopically. Histologically, type II will present with increased intraepithelial lymphocytosis. The villi are typically normal however atrophy may be seen in some cases. Similar to EATL, the prognosis of MEITL is quite poor. Chemotherapy can be used.

Indolent lymphoproliferative disorders of the intestines are clonal proliferations that can be classified as T-cell (CD4+, CD8+, CD4−CD8−), or Natural Killer cell-like. These conditions are not associated with celiac disease and tend to present in adult males. They can be seen throughout the gastrointestinal tract, but are more commonly seen in the small intestine and colon. The disease has an indolent course but can lead to significant symptoms, such as diarrhea, abdominal pain, and weight loss, and can be hard to treat. One recent study found that CD4+ T-cell lymphoproliferative disorders are associated with STAT3-JAK2 fusions. In addition to suggesting a possible pathologic mechanism, this fusion could be used to distinguish lymphoproliferative disorders from reactive processes and may be a target for treatment [24]. Endoscopically, raised lesions (nodules or polypoid), hemorrhages, or ulcers may be seen, either in one location or involving the whole gastrointestinal system. Given the indolent nature, the course is typically chronic. While the risk of lymphoma is low, it has been described in some patients. Histology may show either normal or atrophic villi. Prognosis is good, and typically there is good response to steroids. It is thought that those with the CD4+ phenotype may be at higher risk [25].

NK-cell enteropathy is very rare and again is typically seen around mid-life. There appears to be a female predominance, although this is controversial. Presentation can range from asymptomatic to diarrhea and abdominal pain. The entire gastrointestinal tract is at risk for involvement. NK enteropathy appears to be indolent, and chemotherapy doesn't appear to be effective.

MALT lymphomas typically involve the stomach but can be found anywhere in the gastrointestinal tract. Immunohistochemistry is commonly helpful in identifying this disease, specifically trough a CD20 stain. When the duodenum or jejunum is involved, villous atrophy may be seen.

## Drug/Iatrogenic Enteropathy

Medications are the second most common cause of seronegative villous atrophy after seronegative celiac disease. When investigating the cause of enteropathy, a review of the medication list should be performed early. Diagnosing enteropathy related to medications depends on having a history of taking the drug, having enteropathy either clinically or endoscopically, improvement/resolution with stopping the medication or reducing the dose, and finally excluding alternative causes [26]. Treatment involves withdrawal of the medication if possible. Some medication related enteropathies have more specific therapies, which are detailed below. Mucosal healing is expected around six months after the medication is stopped. A trial off of possible causal medications should be performed early in the investigation of enteropathy if possible.

### Angiotensin Receptor Blockers

Olmesartan is responsible for the majority of cases of enteropathy secondary to medications [27]. The incidence of olmesartan-associated enteropathy is estimated to be 1.3 cases per 1000 individuals per year. Other angiotensin receptor blockers have been implicated in case reports, and suggest that there may be a class effect with these medications, especially the more potent varieties. Individuals have typically been on the medication for years, have autoimmune conditions, and present with severe diarrhea, weight loss, and dehydration that may necessitate hospitalization and total parenteral nutrition [28]. The pathophysiology is thought to be immune-based and involves changes similar to celiac disease including similar cytokines, increased CD8+ cells, and overexpression of IL15 seen in celiac disease [29]. Blood work may show malabsorption, electrolyte abnormalities and hypoalbuminemia [30]. Around 90% will have one of the two permissive haplotypes for celiac disease, HLA-DQ2 or DQ8, however celiac serology will be negative. Histology shows duodenal villous atrophy and intraepithelial lymphocytosis. A thickened subepithelial collagen layer may be seen if collagenous sprue has developed. If individuals are severely ill or slow to respond to respond to drug withdrawal, steroids can be used, such as budesonide 3 mg three times daily.

### Non-steroidal Anti-Inflammatories

Non-steroidal anti-inflammatories (NSAIDs) can cause a number of different complications in the gastrointestinal tract, one of which is enteropathy. The use of video capsule endoscopy has led to increased recognition of this, and it is now thought that up to 70% of those on chronic NSAIDs have small intestinal mucosal injury [31, 32]. Unlike angiotensin receptor blocker associated enteropathy, the enteropathy seen with NSAIDs can develop within weeks of initiation, and has a more subclinical presentation. Weight loss is infrequent, and the most common presentation is one of iron deficiency due to occult bleeding that is estimated to range up to 10 mL of blood per day [31]. The pathophysiology is believed to be multifactorial and includes direct damage, reduced prostaglandin levels leading to increased motility and a compromise of the mucus barrier, and ileal dysbiosis [31]. Concurrent use of proton pump inhibitors, which exacerbates the enteropathy, is thought to do so by worsening this dysbiosis. Laboratory studies are most notable for iron deficiency anemia. Endoscopically, erythema, erosions, and ulcerations may be seen. The degree of damage does not correlate with clinical symptoms. Concentric fibrinous projections in the small intestine (diaphragm strictures) is a pathognomonic finding [31]. If it is not possible to stop the NSAIDs, then the dose should be decreased if possible, or a selective COX-2 inhibitor can be trialed. Additionally, prostaglandin repletion with misoprostol or rebamipide, and addressing dysbiosis with antibiotics or probiotics can also be trialed [31].

## Mycophenolate Mofetil

Mycophenolate mofetil is the most common cause of villous atrophy in the solid organ transplant population [30]. Enteropathy typically develops within one year of being on the medication, and presents with chronic, persistent diarrhea [30]. The enteropathy is thought to be secondary to both direct damage as well as inhibition of purine synthesis causing inhibited cell proliferation. Similar to angiotensin receptor blocker enteropathy, signs of malabsorption and dehydration may be seen in the blood work. While HLA-DQ2 may be seen in nearly 50% of those affected, studies have not found any with HLA-DQ8 [30]. Endoscopically, mucosal erythema, erosions, and ulcerations may be seen, and histology may show crypt dilatation, apoptosis, and an edematous lamina propria. Typically there is no significant intraepithelial lymphocytosis or hyperplasia of the crypts [30]. Stopping immunosuppression with mycophenolate mofetil may not be possible, and in these cases a dose reduction can be trialed and can in some cases leads to symptom resolution [30].

## Methotrexate

Methotrexate, a folic acid antagonist, is used frequently as an immunosuppressive. Rare case-reports detail an association with villous atrophy with symptoms ranging from asymptomatic to malabsorption with diarrhea and weight loss. Labs may show iron deficiency and signs of malabsorption. The pathophysiology is not known, however direct toxicity and a genetic predisposition have been suggested [33, 34].

## Azathioprine

While azathioprine has been frequently used as a steroid sparing agent to treat enteropathy, there have been case reports suggesting that it can be a causal agent as well. These case reports describe severe diarrhea and associated villous atrophy developing within weeks of starting the medication. This villous atrophy extended from the duodenum through the ileum. The afflicted individuals were quite ill, requiring total parenteral nutrition. Symptom resolution occurred within two weeks of stopping the drug, and histologic resolution within four months [30, 35].

## Monoclonal Antibodies

Several monoclonal antibodies have been associated with enteropathy. This includes check point inhibitors, which are increasingly becoming standard practice in oncology. Celiac disease itself has been reported following the use of the checkpoint inhibitors: ipilimumab, a combination of nivolumab and ipilimumab, and possibly pembrolizumab [36–38]. Celiac-like enteropathy has been described with nivolumab. In one of these cases, involvement extended to the colon. These cases presented with severe malabsorption and biopsies showed villous atrophy and intraepithelial lymphocytosis. Celiac serology was negative and there was no response to a gluten-free diet, distinguishing this from the development of celiac disease. The enteropathy developed soon after initiation of nivolumab in one case and in the other after long-term treatment [39].

## Graft-Versus-Host Disease

Graft-versus-host disease (GVHD) complicates up to 40% of allo-hematopoietic stem cell transplants, which are used to treat hematologic diseases, particularly neoplasms. GVHD is subdivided into two separate entities: acute if it occurs within 100 days and chronic if it occurs after 100 days of transplant. Acute and chronic GVHD are distinct, with the former manifesting with epithelial cell death in the skin, intestinal tract, and liver, and the latter involving atrophy and fibrosis of these and other organs.

Acute GVHD is thought to be driven by mature T-lymphocytes in the donor tissue and is associated with significant morbidity and mortality (one study found death in 42%). The development of GVHD also appears to be associated with an altered gut microbiome and loss of bacterial diversity. Likely related to this, the use of broad spectrum antibiotics has been found to be associated with the development of intestinal GVHD [40]. The conditioning needed prior to transplantation is thought to initiate intestinal GVHD, with continued intestinal barrier loss propagating the disease [41]. The skin is most commonly involved, followed by the intestines, and liver. Acute intestinal GVID typically presents with severe diarrhea three weeks after transplant, although dyspepsia, nausea, and vomiting can also be seen.

Typically, intestinal involvement mirrors skin and liver involvement, so individuals will likely (but not always) have jaundice and a rash. Diagnosis relies on biopsies, either of the intestine, stomach, colon, liver, or skin. The highest yield biopsies for intestinal GVHD appear to be those from the right colon, terminal ileum, and duodenum. Both endoscopically normal and abnormal tissue should be biopsied. The degree of atrophy in the biopsies from the terminal ileum in particular is predictive of the severity of the disease and the likelihood for it to be steroid resistant. Opportunistic infections, which are common, can mimic acute GVHD and need to be excluded. Common intestinal infections include astrovirus, clostridium difficile, and adenovirus. Endoscopy commonly shows gross abnormalities in roughly 50% of cases. This includes erosions, ulcers, gastritis, and subepithelial hemorrhage. Biopsies from the duodenum will show villous atrophy, cell vacuolization, and a granulomononuclear inflammatory infiltrate [42]. Apoptotic bodies can also be seen. The presence of severe crypt loss has been associated with disease severity.

Chronic GVHD involves fibrosis and immunodeficiency, and in the majority of cases is preceded by acute GVHD. Chronic GVHD occurs in 30 to 70% of individuals, and can involve any organ system. However, intestinal chronic GVHD is thought to be uncommon, with one study estimating an incidence of 7.3% [43]. Risk factors for chronic GVHD include having acute GVHD, older age, chronic myeloid leukemia, and sex and HLA disparities between the donor and recipient. Chronic GVHD is thought to have several steps in development: tissue injury leading to inflammation, development of chronic inflammation and dysregulated B and T cell immunity leading to tissue repair and fibrosis. Most patients are symptomatic and present with diarrhea, nausea, vomiting, and malabsorption which in some cases requires total parenteral nutrition. Most commonly several additional organs are involved and can include in order of decreasing frequency, skin, liver, and lung. Previously, diagnosis was challenging due to the number of different manifestations, however in 2005 the NIH developed a criteria for diagnosis as well as a risk score that has helped standardize approach to this condition. Endoscopically, the mucosa typically appears normal or can have some slight erythema. Histology can show glandular epithelial apoptosis, sparse diffuse inflammatory infiltrate, and villous atrophy in 60% of those tested in one study. Most patients do get treated with an immunosuppressive, typically for several years, and symptom resolution occurred in nearly 60%.

Prophylaxis against acute GVHD includes the use of cyclosporine and methotrexate or mycophenolate mofetil. Due to its impact on the thymus and T-regulatory cell function, cyclosporine may increase the risk for chronic GVHD. Anti-T cell globulin and high dose cyclophosphamide may help prevent chronic GVHD, however anti-T cell globulin has been associated with a significantly increased risk of death. Recent studies have been investigating the use of vedolizumab as a prophylactic medication [44].

For both acute and chronic GVHD, steroids are the first line of therapy, and supportive cares including nutritional, fluids, and electrolytes are crucial. Steroids should include both systemic steroids and oral minimally absorbable steroids, such as beclomethasone and budesonide. The use of minimally absorbed steroids has been found to increase responsiveness and to allow tapering of systemic steroids.

Resistance to steroids suggests a very poor prognosis, with only 30% surviving in five years. There is no standard second-line therapy for steroid resistant GVHD, however there have been many medications that have been tested. For acute GVHD, options include alpha-1 antitrypsin, antithymocyte globulin, interleukin-2 receptor (CD25alpha) antibodies, alemtuzumab, brentuximab, tocilizumab, daclizumab, mycophenolate mofetil, etanercept, pentostatin, ruxolitinib, sirolimus, and extracorporeal photophoresis. For chronic GVHD, options include cyclosporine, tacrolimus, mycophenolate mofetil, thalidomide, hydroxychloroquine, methotrexate, rituximab, ibrutinib, and others. Blood stream infections have been associated with intestinal GVHD, which is thought to be secondary to bacterial translocation.

## Chemotherapy

Chemotherapy is known to damage mucous membranes, leading to mild gastrointestinal mucositis in 15% of individuals and severe in 2% [45]. Mucositis is a significant complication of chemotherapy, as it can lead to significant morbidity, mortality, delayed chemotherapy, and increased health care costs [46]. Symptoms include diarrhea, abdominal pain, and malabsorption. The National Institute of Health (NIH) has developed a scoring system to assess the severity of diarrhea, ranging from Grade I (an increase of less than four stools per day) to grade five (death). The enteropathy is postulated to be secondary to the impact of chemotherapy on the high turnover of cells in the small intestine. The initialization phase results from direct cell injury either from DNA damage or reactive oxygen species. This triggers an inflammatory response in which immunoglobulin A plays an important protective role. This inflammation triggers further damage and impacts the intestinal barrier, leading to increased translocation of bacteria. Apoptosis in intestinal crypts has been observed one day following chemotherapy. At three days, enterocyte height, villous area, and crypt length were found to have decreased, and by 16 days post-chemotherapy these changes had improved [47]. The risk of mucositis is related to the specific chemotherapy used. Agents known to cause intestinal mucositis include: irinotecan, fluoropyrimidines (including 5-FU), paclitaxel, oxaliplatin, lapatinib, methotrexate, taxanes, cisplatin, carboplatin. The risk for and severity of mucositis is related to the regimen being used. Some of the biggest offenders are irinotecan and 5-FU, which when given weekly cause 10% of patients to develop severe mucositis. Oral immunoglobulin A may help decrease the risk of intestinal mucositis. There is no targeted therapy for this condition, and treatment is therefore supportive. Avoidance of foods associated with diarrhea and emphasizing hydration, and medications such as loperamide, octreotide, activated charcoal, and probiotics can be used (although the evidence in support is often poor) [48].

## Radiation

Similar to chemotherapy, radiation can also lead to mucositis and associated diarrhea, abdominal pain, nausea, vomiting, and malabsorption. Pelvic radiotherapy can lead to diarrhea in up to 90% of patients and mucositis in 50%. Diarrhea can result not only from mucositis but also from altered intestinal motility, alterations in the microbiome, bile-acid malabsorption, and secondary lactose intolerance. Radiation is thought to cause mucositis through direct injury to the epithelium, inflammation, and tissue ischemia, resulting in villous blunting. Damage can be seen histologically within hours of receiving radiation therapy, however symptoms typically occur after three weeks of therapy. Risk factors for radiation-induced intestinal mucositis include patient age, total radiation dose, receiving radiation in the morning, the amount of tissue irradiated, and the fractionation schedule [49]. Concurrent chemotherapy also appears to increase the risk. Again, there is no targeted therapy aside from symptomatic management. Resolution of symptoms typically occurs within six weeks of stopping radiation therapy.

## *Infectious Enteropathy*

### Giardiasis

The protozoa *Giardia lamblia* (or *duodenalis*) is one of the most common causes of infectious gastroenteritis worldwide, and is particularly common in developing countries. The parasite is transmitted through a fecal-oral route via ingestion of the infectious cysts. The infectious dose may be as little as 10 cysts, and the incubation period is between 9 and 15 days. The protozoa adhere to the intestinal epithelium and are thought to disrupt epithelial cell junctions and brush border enzymes. This in turn leads to increased intestinal permeability and a loss of ability to process saccharides. Villous atrophy in the setting of giardiasis infection was first noted in 1978 [50]. Mucosal changes can vary from normal to total villous atrophy, and the severity of atrophy appears to have a direct relationship with the severity of symptoms [51]. One case-series found that roughly 62% had villous atrophy, 64% had increased intraepithelial lymphocytes and 43.3% had lymphoid follicles [52]. Another study on a pediatric population found a much lower rate of villous atrophy (3%) [53].

High-risk groups include men who have sex with men, those who travel or visit the wilderness, daycare workers, and people who come into contact with human feces. While somewhat controversial, immunoglobulin A (IgA) deficiency is believed to be a risk factor, and IgA has been found to play a significant role in eradication of the infection [54]. Symptoms can range from being none (~50%—carriers) to severe watery diarrhea, fat malabsorption, abdominal pain, and weight loss [55]. Symptoms typically self-resolve in four weeks, however chronic infections can develop. The infection can be diagnosed with stool antigen detection assays and nucleic acid amplification tests. Microscopy can be performed but because the protozoa are only intermittently shed, this may not be successful in identification. Metronidazole is the first line treatment, and typically is given as 250 to 500 mg three times daily for 5 to 10 days. One study found that mucosal abnormalities resolved within one month of treatment [55].

## Whipple's Disease

Whipple's disease is rare (estimated prevalence of three in 1,000,000) and secondary to a gram-positive, rod shaped bacteria, *Tropheryma whipplei*, that is prevalent in the environment, specifically sewage water [56]. Given the prevalence of the bacteria, but rarity of the disease, it is postulated that there may be host, pathogen, and environmental factors that impact susceptibility. A genetic predisposition has been suggested. With exposure, individuals can have an acute or chronic infection, or become carriers. Carriers are believed to be a significant reservoir, and high-risk groups include sewage workers, the homeless, those with a family member with Whipple's disease, and cirrhotics [57–60]. The disease classically affects middle-aged males.

Transmission is believed to be fecal-oral, oral-oral, and potentially respiratory. *Tropheryma whipplei* utilizes the host's immune system for its replication and propagation. Macrophages internalize the bacteria which ultimately induce apoptosis, releasing replicated bacteria into the tissue.

Symptoms of Whipple's disease are varied. Acute infection can present as pneumonia, bacteremia, and gastroenteritis. The symptoms of localized infection are determined by which tissue is involved, but require an absence of gut and systemic involvement [61]. Classic Whipple's disease (a chronic systemic infection) has been described as presenting with a characteristic combination of fever, diarrhea, abdominal pain, and arthralgias. However, one recent case-series found that the presence of all four symptoms is in fact rare [61]. Infection manifests in three stages: early, middle, and late [56]. The early phase is marked by acute inflammatory attacks with fever and arthralgias. This then progresses to diarrhea and weight loss (middle phase), and finally to systemic symptoms involving the central nervous system, eyes, and heart (late phase). Common symptoms include weight loss, diarrhea, adenopathy, fever, neurologic symptoms, and arthritis. Oculomasticatory myorhythmia is a pathognomonic but rare finding.

Diagnosis can be difficult, and this condition is often misdiagnosed. Laboratory findings may show microcytic anemia and elevated inflammatory markers. The gross appearance on upper endoscopy is most often normal. Because the disease has a patchy distribution, multiple biopsies should be obtained from the duodenum, gastric antrum, jejunum, and ileum if possible. Histopathology using a Periodic acid-Schiff (PAS) stain will identify PAS-positive foamy macrophages in the lamina propria [62]. This is a non-specific finding, however, and a Ziehl-Neelsen stain can be used to distinguish this from mycobacterial infections [63]. PCR and immunohistochemistry can also be performed on the biopsy specimens. Biopsies should undergo at least two modalities of testing: PAS staining as well as either PCR and or immunohistochemistry. Positive PAS staining and either PCR or immunohisto-chemistry or PAS negative but positive PCR and immunohistochemistry all confirm Whipple's disease. If only one of these three tests return positive, this connotes possible Whipple's disease, and further testing should be considered. Additional testing includes saliva and stool PCR, serology, fluorescence *in situ* hybridization, and electron microscopy [56].

Treatment is somewhat controversial. One regimen involves ceftriaxone (two grams/day) for 14 days followed by oral trimethoprim-sulfamethoxazole (160 mg/800 mg per day) for one year. However, there is growing concern that *Tropheryma whipplei* is resistant to trimethoprim-sulfamethoxazole, and an alternative regimen involves doxycycline (200 mg/day) and hydroxychloroquine (600 mg/day) for 12 months followed by maintenance doxycycline for life. Relapses are common and when these involve the central nervous system, prognosis is poor.

## Human Immunodeficiency Virus

The *Human Immunodeficiency Virus* (HIV) can cause villous atrophy in roughly 50% of those infected, regardless of disease stage [64]. This is independent of opportunistic infections. In acute HIV infection, there is infiltration of the gastrointestinal mucosa with activated effector memory CD4+ and CD8+ T-cells and the epithelial barrier is impaired [65]. This is then followed by severe depletion of the CD4+ T-cells in the mucosa (particularly Th17 cells) [66, 67]. Histologically, this is characterized by partial villous atrophy with crypt hyperproliferation and villous shortening [64]. Severe atrophy is rarely seen, and the extent of atrophy is similar to celiac disease [64]. Roughly 80% of those with villous atrophy will be symptomatic with diarrhea, however notably, the prevalence of diarrhea in those with villous atrophy was not significantly different than the prevalence in those without [64]. This is likely related to the high frequency of diarrhea in those with HIV. Medication side-effects and opportunistic infections need to be tested for [68]. HIV enteropathy has potentially significant implications, as the defect in the intestinal barrier is thought to lead to microbial translocation and systemic inflammation that in turn leads to complications such as cardiovascular disease [69, 70]. While highly active antiretroviral therapy (HAART) is crucial in HIV, its impact on enteropathy is delayed [66, 67]. Studies have found that the restoration of the intestinal T-cell population after HAART initiation can be slow and incomplete. The process does appear to occur more quickly when HAART is initiated early in the infection [66]. The repopulation of the mucosa seems to be secondary to cell trafficking as opposed to local proliferation. One recent randomized double blind study suggests that oral serum-derived bovine immunoglobulin/protein isolate may help support gut healing and decrease systemic inflammation [69].

## Tropical Sprue

Tropical sprue has an estimated incidence of 0.24 per 100,000 person-years, affects men and women equally, and typically presents in people in their mid-30s [71]. The disease is seen in India, South east Asia, the Caribbean, Central America and Africa, Mexico, Venezuela, and Columbia. Although rarely seen in Europe and North America, it can affect travelers and military personnel deployed to affected countries, as well as expatriates. A significant risk factor for tropical sprue is prior infectious gastroenteritis (odds ratio of 34.6, 95% confidence intervals 4.8–282.4) [72]. A history of travel can help distinguish tropical sprue from celiac disease. Although not certain, tropical sprue is believed to be an infectious disease. This is supported by the association with prior infectious gastroenteritis, by reported epidemics, the positive response to antibiotics, and the association with small intestinal bacterial overgrowth. Symptoms involve chronic diarrhea, abdominal pain and bloating, fatigue, weight loss, fever, and steatorrhea [73, 74]. While some cases can undergo remission, others can lead to severe malnutrition and even death.

Diagnosis of tropical sprue requires five criteria be met: 1) an appropriate clinical presentation (to distinguish from the more common environmental enteropathy) 2) malabsorption of two unrelated substances, 3) abnormal small intestinal histology 4) exclusion of other possible disease processes (not including small intestinal bacterial overgrowth) and 5) response to appropriate treatment. Laboratory testing can show the classic findings of vitamin B12 and folate deficiency. Anti-gliadin antibodies are common in tropical sprue, but other celiac serologies should be absent. Upper endoscopy commonly shows duodenal scalloping, and the small bowel histology is indistinguishable from that seen in celiac disease [71, 73]. Tropical sprue can involve the entire small bowel, and commonly involves the terminal ileum. Treatment is folic acid (5 mg daily) in combination with tetracycline (250 mg four times daily) for three to six months. Relapse can be seen in one in five individuals.

## Small Intestinal Bacterial Overgrowth

Small intestinal bacterial overgrowth (SIBO) is characterized by elevated bacterial levels in the small intestine accompanied by gastrointestinal symptoms. The prevalence of SIBO is not known as diagnosis relies on specialized procedures. There have been numerous risk factors identified that include female sex, increasing age, proton-pump inhibitors, opioids, surgical interventions (gastric bypass, colectomy, hysterectomy, cholecystectomy), dysmotility, inflammatory bowel disease, small bowel diverticula, pancreatitis, hypothyroidism, coronary artery disease, diabetes, and Parkinson's [75, 76]. While celiac disease is believed to be a risk factor, some studies question this association [77]. Symptoms include in order of decreasing prevalence: diarrhea, weight loss, abdominal pain, and abdominal bloating [78]. However, the presence of symptoms cannot identify those with SIBO versus those without [75, 79]. The gold standard diagnostic test is small bowel aspirates/culture with a growth of over $10^3$ colony forming unit (CFU)/mL being a positive result (some suggest using $10^5$ CFU/mL as a threshold) [80]. This test does have risks for a false-positive result secondary to contamination by oral flora. A glucose or lactulose breath test can also be performed, however this test has poor sensitivity and specificity and is impacted by recent medication use such as antibiotics and prokinetics, as well as recent diet, smoking, and physical activity [80, 81]. While more than half of small bowel biopsies from those with SIBO are unremarkable, roughly 24% can show villous atrophy [78]. Treatment is with antibiotic courses. Rifaximin is one frequently used antibiotic due to its safety profile and efficacy [82]. Other antibiotics include ciprofloxacin, norfloxacin, and metronidazole. Probiotics appear to help with clearance of SIBO but not prevention [83]. It is estimated that 44% of individuals will have recurrent SIBO despite antibiotic therapy, and up to 40% will have treatment failures. A lack of response of symptoms to treatment may suggest either another underlying cause for the symptoms versus antibiotic resistant bacteria. The initial approach to recurrent SIBO involves small bowel aspiration and culture in order to identify the culprit bacteria and target therapy. Additionally, if any risk factors are identified, they could be ameliorated—for instance, by discontinuing opioids. Prokinetics could be considered but this approach has little evidence. For individuals with a risk factor which cannot be resolved, cyclic antibiotic courses can be implemented.

## Collagenous Sprue

Collagenous sprue is a rare enteropathy that classically has been viewed as a complication of celiac disease, and often refractory celiac disease. There is an increasing recognition of additional triggering factors, including drugs such as olmesartan and non-steroidal anti-inflammatories [84–86]. Individuals with collagenous sprue are often elderly, although recent case-reports have been described in infants. It appears to be more common in females, is frequently associated with immune-mediated disorders, and more than half of individuals are on medications such as non-steroidal anti-inflammatories, proton-pump inhibitors, or olmesartan.

The pathophysiology is not fully understood, but it is thought to be immune mediated. Increased IgG4 positive plasma cells have been seen and are thought to contribute to disease progression. It is postulated that there are environmental triggers like drugs (in particular olmesartan and non-steroidal anti-inflammatories), gluten, food antigens, or infections that may trigger development of collagenous sprue [87].

Typical symptoms include chronic diarrhea, malabsorption, and weight loss (one study reports a median weight loss of 27 pounds). Laboratory studies may show anemia and hypoalbuminemia. Some individuals may be endomysial antibody positive and have signs of hyposplenism [88]. Histologically, collagenous sprue presents with villous atrophy, intraepithelial lymphocytes, and subepithelial collagen. There is no cut off collagen thickness needed to make the diagnosis, however one study found that the average thickness was 29 micrometers. The distribution of collagen is most commonly diffuse, but in 25% can be patchy. The presence of clonal T-cells has been identified in some studies, but not others [89]. Individuals with collagenous sprue frequently will also have collagenous gastritis or colitis.

The prognosis has generally been viewed as poor and the need for total parenteral nutrition is common [90]. Steroids are commonly used, including prednisone and budesonide. A gluten-free diet is only effective in some individuals (one study estimated 42%), and a combination of this and steroids is often recommended [84]. Azathioprine has been used as a steroid sparing agent, and one case-report found good response to infliximab [91]. Complete remission is possible. Possible but infrequent complications include small bowel ulceration, lymphoma, and perforation [84].

## Eosinophilic Gastroenteritis

First described in 1937, eosinophilic gastroenteritis is a rare condition with an estimated prevalence in the United States of 8.4–28/100,000 [92, 93]. The diagnosis rests on three criteria: 1) the presence of gastrointestinal symptoms 2) eosinophilic infiltration of gastrointestinal mucosa or the presence of eosinophilic ascites and 3) exclusion of alternative etiologies [94]. There are three subgroups based on anatomic involvement: mucosal (up to 100% of cases), muscular (up to 70% of cases), and serosal (up to 13% of cases) [94, 95]. The colon and esophagus can be involved in addition to the stomach and small intestine. Risk factors appear to be younger age (highest prevalence in those below five years of age), atopic conditions (seen in 45.6% of cases), living in the South and Midwest of the US, having a family history of atopic conditions (suggesting a genetic tie), higher socioeconomic status, Caucasian race, celiac disease, and ulcerative colitis [92, 96–98]. Unlike eosinophilic gastritis, there does not appear to be a sex predominance [92]. The cause of eosinophilic gastroenteritis is not yet fully understood. Given the associated atopic and immune-related conditions, it is hypothesized that the condition may be secondary to an allergic reaction triggering immune dysregulation. Environmental triggering factors have been proposed and include drugs and parasites. Multiple chemokines and mediators, including interleukin-5 recruit eosinophils to the gastrointestinal tract where they in turn release their own mediators, causing inflammation and damage to the intestine. Because the muscular and serosal subtypes are associated with the mucosal, a centrifugal progression has been proposed.

The symptoms of eosinophilic gastroenteritis in order of decreasing prevalence include abdominal pain/dyspepsia, diarrhea, nausea/vomiting, and chest pain [92]. Protein-losing enteropathy and malabsorption can be seen. If the muscular layer is involved, bowel wall thickening and intestinal obstruction may be observed, and if the infiltration extends to the serosa, ascites with a high eosinophil count may be present as well as peritonitis and perforation. Laboratory studies may show anemia and hypoalbuminemia [99]. Peripheral eosinophilia is common but not necessary (one study reported up to 72%) [99]. Elevated IgE can be seen as well [99]. Radiographic findings can be normal in up to 40%, or can identify thickened intestinal wall and mucosal folds [100].

Endoscopic findings are non-specific and include ulceration, erythema, pseudo-polyps, and polyps [99]. Because the disease has a patchy distribution, multiple biopsies, at least five, need to be obtained from both normal and abnormal appearing mucosa [101]. If muscular involvement is suspected, endoscopic ultrasound with fine needle aspiration can be utilized for biopsies. Biopsies can show villous atrophy, crypt hyperplasia, as well as eosinophilic infiltrates [102]. Normal eosinophil levels vary depending on age and location in the gastrointestinal tract. Normal eosinophil levels in the duodenum for adults is less than 19, so 20 eosinophils per high-power field (hpf) is considered the threshold for gastroenteritis. Other disorders that cause elevated eosinophils need to be evaluated for and ruled out (such as intestinal parasites with stool testing, celiac disease, idiopathic hypereosinophilic syndrome, and inflammatory bowel disease).

Spontaneous remission can be seen in up to 40% of cases, a flare followed by remission in 42%, multiple flares in 37% separated by full remission, and 21% with chronic disease [103]. The mainstay of treatment is steroids such as prednisolone and budesonide. Dietary therapy involving either a targeted elimination diet based on identified allergens, a standard six or seven food elimination diet, or the elemental diet can also be used but is controversial. Other treatments include leukotriene receptor antagonists, mast cell stabilizers, antihistamines, immunomodulators, proton pump inhibitors, biologic agents, IVIG, interferon alpha, and fecal microbiota transplant. Duration of therapy and whether to instate maintenance therapy is controversial, and solid evidence on the efficacy of most treatments is lacking (Table 1).

**Table 1** Histologic features and geographical distribution of conditions that can cause severe enteropathy and villous atrophy

| Condition | Histology | | | Geographic Distribution | | | | |
|---|---|---|---|---|---|---|---|---|
| | Villous Atrophy | Intraepithelial lymphocytosis | Additional findings on histology | Stomach | Duodenum | Ileum | Jejunum | Colon |
| Environmental Enteropathy | + | + | None | | | | | |
| Autoimmune Enteropathy | + | - | Paneth and Goblet cells may be absent | | | | | |
| Common variable immunodeficiency enteropathy | + | + | *Absence of plasma cells *Lymphoid nodular hyperplasia *Crohn's like or Graft-versus-host-like lesions *Polymorphonuclear infiltrate *Apoptotic cells | | | | | |
| Lymphoproliferative Disorders | + | + | Type 1 EATL: CD3+, CD4-, CD5-, CD7+, CD8-, CD30+, CD56-, CD103+, TCR$\beta$+ Type 2 EATL: CD3+, CD4-, CD8+, CD30-, CD56+, TCR$\beta$+ MALT: CD20+ B cells and plasma cells with $\alpha$ heavy chain but no light chains | | | | | |
| Angiotensin receptor blockers | + | + | None | | | | | |
| Graft-versus-host disease | +/- | + | Granulomononuclear inflmammatory infiltrate and apoptotic bodies | | | | | |
| Chemotherapy | + | + | None | | | | | |
| Radiation | + | + | None | | | | | |
| Giardiasis | +/- | +/- | May show lymphoid follicles | | | | | |
| Whipple's Disease | + | + | Periodic acid-Schiff (PAS) stain positive diastase – macrophage infiltration in lamina propria | | | | | |
| HIV | + | + | None | | | | | |
| Tropical Sprue | + | + | None | | | | | |
| Small intestinal bacterial overgrowth | +/- | + | None | | | | | |
| Collagenous Sprue | + | + | Subepithelial collagen band | | | | | |
| Eosinophilic gastroenteritis | + | - | Eosinophilic infiltration (>20 per high-power field) | | | | | |

# References

1. Amadi B, Besa E, Zyambo K, Kaonga P, Louis-Auguste J, Chandwe K, et al. Impaired barrier function and autoantibody generation in malnutrition enteropathy in Zambia. EBioMedicine. 2017;22:191–9.
2. Guerrant R, DeBoer M, Moore S, Scharf R, Lima A. The impoverished gut - a triple burden of diarrhoea, stunting and chronic disease. Nat Rev Gastroenterol Hepatol. 2013;10:220–9.
3. Platts-Mills J, Babji S, Bodhidatta L, Gratz J, Haque R, Havt A, et al. Pathogen-specific burdens of community diarrhoea in developing countries: a multisite bortih cohort study (MAL-ED). Lancet Glob Health. 2015;3(9):e564–75.
4. Dewey K, Adu-Afarwuah S. Systematic review of the efficacy and effectiveness of complementary feeding interventions in developing countries. Matern Child Nutr. 2008;4:24–85.
5. Bhutta Z, Ahmed T, Black R, Cousens S, Dewey K, Giugliani E, et al. What works? Interventions for maternal and child undernutrition and survival. Lancet. 2008;371:417–40.

6. Levine M. Immunogenicity and efficacy of oral vaccines in developing countries: lessons from a live cholera vaccine. BMC Biol. 2010;8:129.
7. Campbell D, Murch S, Elia M, Sullivan P, Sanyang M, Jobarteh B, et al. Chronic T cell-mediated enteropathy in rural West African children: relationship with nutritional status and small bowel function. Pediatr Res. 2003;54(3):306–11.
8. Akram S, Murray J, Pardi D, Alexander G, Schaffner J, Russo P, et al. Adult autoimmune enteropathy: Mayo Clinic Rochester experience. Clin Gastroenterol Hepatol. 2007 Nov;5(11):1282–90.
9. Sharma A, Choung R, Wang X, Russo P, Wu T, Nehra V, et al. Features of adult autoimmune enteropathy compared with refractory celiac disease. Clin Gastroenterol Hepatol. 2018;16(6):877–83.e1.
10. Mais D, Mulhall B, Adolphson K, Yamamoto K. Thymoma-associated autoimmune enteropathy. A report of two cases. Am J Clin Pathol. 1999;112(6):810–5.
11. Umetsu S, Brown I, Langner C, Lauwers G. Autoimmune enteropathies. Virchows Arch. 2018;472(1):55–66.
12. Duclaux-Loras R, Charbit-Henrion F, Neven B, Nowak J, Collardeau-Frachon S, Malcus C, et al. Clinical heterogeneity of immune dysregulation, polyendocrinopathy, enteropathy, X-linked syndrome: a French multicenter retrospective study. Clin Transl Gastroenterol. 2018;9(10):201.
13. Parlato M, Charbit-Henrion F, Abi Nader E, Begue B, Guegan N, Bruneau J, et al. Efficacy of ruxolitinib therapy in a patient with severe enterocolitis associated with a STAT3 gain-of-function mutation. Gastroenterology. 2019;156(4):1206–10.
14. Charbit-Henrion F, Jeverica A, Begue B, Markelj G, Parlato M, Avcin S, et al. Deficiency in mucosa-associated lymphoid tissue lymphoma translocation 1: a novel cause of IPEX-like syndrome. J Pediatr Gastroenterol Nutr. 2017;64(3):378–84.
15. Boland B, Widjaja C, Banno A, Zhang B, Kim S, Stoven S, et al. Immunodeficiency and autoimmune enterocolopathy linked to NFAT5 haploinsufficiency. J Immunol. 2015;195(6):2551–60.
16. Lei A, Azhari H, Raman M. A117 a case of adult autoimmune enteropathy and primary sclerosing cholangitis. J Can Assoc Gastroenterol. 2020;3(Supplement_1):135–7.
17. Malamut G, Verkarre V, Suarez F, Viallard J, Lascaux A-S, Cosnes J, et al. The enteropathy associated with common variable immunodeficiency: the delineated frontiers with celiac disease. Am J Gastroenterol. 2010;105(10):2262–75.
18. Martinez-Gallo M, Radigan L, Almejun M, Martinez-Pomar N, Matamoros N, Cunningham-Rundles C. TACI mutations and impaired B-cell function in subjects with CVID and healthy heterozygotes. J Allergy Clin Immunol. 2012;131(2):468–76.
19. Biagi F, Bianchi P, Zilli A, Marchese A, Luinetti O, Lougaris V, et al. The significance of duodenal mucosal atrophy in patients with common variable immunodeficiency: a clinical and histopathologic study. Am J Clin Pathol. 2012;138(2):185–9.
20. Venhoff N, Emmerich F, Neagu M, Salzer U, Koehn C, Driever S, et al. The role of HLA DQ2 and DQ8 in dissecting celiac-like disease in common variable immunodeficiency. J Clin Immunol. 2013;33(5):909–16.
21. Cunningham-Rundles C. How I treat common variable immune deficiency. Blood. 2010;116(1):7–15.
22. Skinnider B. Lymphoproliferative disorders of the gastrointestinal tract. Arch Pathol Lab Med. 2018;142:44–52.
23. Van Vliet C, Spagnolo D. T- and NK-cell lymphoproliferative disorders of the gastrointestinal tract: review and update. Pathology. 2020;52(1):128–41.
24. Sharma A, Oishi N, Boddicker R, Hu G, Benson H, Ketterling R, et al. Recurrent STAT3-JAK2 fusions in indolent T-cell lymphoproliferative disorder of the gastrointestinal tract. Blood. 2018;131(20):2262–6.
25. Matnani R, Ganapathi K, Lewis S, Green P, Alobeid B, Bhagat G. Indolent T- and NK-cell lymphoproliferative disorders of the gastrointestinal tract: a review and update. Hematol Oncol. 2017;35(1):3–16.

26. Hujoel I, Rubio-Tapia A. Sprue-like enteropathy associated with olmesartan: a new kid on the enteropathy block. GE Port J Gastroenterol. 2016 Mar;23(2):61–5.
27. DeGaetani M, Tennyson C, Lebwohl B, Lewis S, Abu Daya H, Arguelles-Grande C, et al. Villous atrophy and negative celiac serology: a diagnostic and therapeutic dilemma. Am J Gastroenterol. 2013 May;108(5):647–53.
28. Rubio-Tapia A, Herman M, Ludvigsson J, Kelly D, Mangan T, Wu T, et al. Severe spruelike enteropathy associated with olmesartan. Mayo Clin Proc. 2012 Aug;87(8):732–8.
29. Marietta E, Nadeau A, Cartee A, Singh I, Rishi A, Choung R, et al. Immunopathogenesis of olmesartan-associated enteropathy. Aliment Pharmacol Ther. 2015 Dec;42(11):1303–14.
30. Weclawiak H, Ould-Mohamed A, Bournet B, Guilbeau-Frugier C, Fortenfant F, Muscari F, et al. Duodenal villous atrophy: a cause of chronic diarrhea after solid-organ transplantation. Am J Transplant. 2011 Mar;11(3):575–82.
31. Tai F, McAlindon M. NSAIDs and the small bowel. Curr Opin Gastroenterol. 2018 May;34(3):175–82.
32. Shin S, Noh C, Lim S, Lee K, Lee K. Non-steroidal anti-inflammatory drug-induced enteropathy. Intest Res. 2017;15(4):446–55.
33. Bosca M, Anon R, Mayordomo E, Villagrasa R, Balza N, Amoros C, et al. Methotreate induced sprue-like syndrome. World J Gastroenterol. 2008;14(45):7009–11.
34. Houtman P, Hofstra S, Spoelstra P. Non-coeliac sprue possibly related to methotrexate in a rheumatoid arthritis patient. Neth J Med. 1995;47(3):113–6.
35. Ziegler T, Fernandez-Estivariz C, Gu L, Fried M, Leader L. Severe villus atrophy and chronic malabsorption induced by azathioprine. Gastroenterology. 2003;124:1950–7.
36. Gentile N, D'Souza A, Fujii L, Wu T, Murray J. Association between ipilimumab and celiac disease. Mayo Clin Proc. 2013;88(4):414–7.
37. Arnouk J, Mathew D, Nulton E, Rachakonda V. A celiac disease phenotype after checkpoint inhibitor exposure: an example of immune dysregulation after immunotherapy. ACG Case Rep J. 2019;6:1–3.
38. Alsaadi D, Shah N, Charabaty A, Atkins M. A case of checkpoint inhibitor-induced celiac disease. J Immunother Cancer. 2019;7:203.
39. Duval L, Habes S, Chatellier T, Guerzider P, Bossard C, Masliah C, et al. Nivolumab-induced celiac-like enteropathy in patient with metastatic renal cell carcinoma: case report and review of the literature. Clin Case Rep. 2019;7:1689–93.
40. Staffas A, Burgos da Silva M, van den Brink M. The intestinal microbiota in allogeneic hematopoietic cell transplant and graft-versus-host disease. Blood. 2017;129(8):927–33.
41. Nalle S, Zuo L, Ong M, Singh G, Worthylake A, Choi W, et al. Graft-versus-host disease propagation depends on increased intestinal epithelial tight junction permeability. J Clin Invest. 2019;129(2):902–14.
42. Borges L, Vilela E, Ferrari M, Cunha A, Vasconcelos A, Torres H. Diagnosis of acute graft-versus-host disease in the gastrointestinal tract of patietns undergoing allogeneic hematopoietic stem cell transplantation. A descriptive and critical study of diagnostic tests. Hematol Transfus Cell Ther. 2020;42(3):245–51.
43. de Serre N, Reijasse D, Verkarre V, Canioni D, Colomb V, Haddad E, et al. Chronic intestinal graft-versus-host disease: clinical, histological and immunohistochemical analysis of 17 children. Bone Marrow Transplant. 2002;29:223–30.
44. Chen Y, Shah N, Renteria A, Cutler C, Jansson J, Akbari M, et al. Vedolizumab for prevention of gravt-versus-host disease after allogeneic hematopoietic stem cell transplantation. Blood Adv. 2019;3(23):4136–46.
45. Jones J, Avritscher E, Cooksley C, Michelet M, Bekele B, Elting L. Epidemiology of treatment-associated mucosal injury after treatment with newer regimens for lymphoma, breast, lung, or colorectal cancer. Support Care Cancer. 2006;14(6):505–15.
46. Dranitsaris G, Maroun J, Shah A. Severe chemotherapy-induced diarrhea in patients with colorectal cancer: a cost of illness analysis. Support Care Cancer. 2005;13(5):318–24.
47. Keefe D, Brealey J, Goland G, Cummins A. Chemotherapy for cancer causes apoptosis that precedes hypoplasia in crypts of the small intestine in humans. Gut. 2000;47(5):632–7.

48. Ribeiro R, Wanderley C, Wong D, Mota J, Leite C, Souza M, Cunha FQ, et al. Irinotecan- and 5-fluorouracil-induced intestinal mucositis: insights into pathogenesis and therapeutic perspectives. Cancer Chemother Pharmacol. 2016;78:881–93.

49. Shukla P, Gupta D, Bisht S, Pant M, Bhatt M, Gupta R, et al. Circadian variation in radiation-induced intestinal mucositis in patients with cervical carcinoma. Cancer. 2010;116(8):2031–5.

50. Levinson J, Nastro L. Giardiasis with total villous atrophy. Gastroenterology. 1978;74(2 Pt 1):271–5.

51. Duncombe V, Bolin T, Davis A, Cummins A, Crouch R. Histopathology in giardiasis: a correlation with diarrhoea. Aust NZ J Med. 1978;8(4):392–6.

52. Arevalo F, Aragon V, Morales L, Morales Caramutti D, Arandia J, Alcocer G. Duodenal villous atrophy, an unexpectedly common finding in giardia lamblia infestation. Rev Gastroenterol Peru. 2010;30(4):272–6.

53. Koot B, ten Kate F, Juffrie M, Rosalina I, Taminiau J, Benninga M. Does giardia lamblia cause villous atrophy in children?: a retrospective cohort study of the histological abnormalities in giardiasis. J Pediatr Gastroenterol Nutr. 2009;49(3):304–8.

54. Langford D, Housley M, Boes M, Chen J, Kagnoff M, Gillin F, et al. Central importance of immunoglobulin a in host defense against *Giardia* spp. Infect Immun. 2002;70(1):11–8.

55. Gillon J. Clinical studies in adults presenting with giardiasis to a gastrointestinal unit. Scott Med J. 1985;30(2):89–95.

56. Dolmans R, Boel C, Lacle M, Kusters J. Clinical manifestations, treatment, and diagnosis of tropheryma whipplei infections. Clin Microbiol Rev. 2017;30(2):529–55.

57. Fenollar F, Trani M, Davoust B, Salle B, Birg M, Rolain J, et al. Prevalence of asymptomatic tropheryma whipplei carriage among humans and nonhuman primates. J Infect Dis. 2008;197(6):880–7.

58. Schoniger-Hekele M, Petermann D, Weber B, Muller C. Tropheryma whipplei in the environment: survey of sewage plant influxes and sewage plant workers. Appl Environ Microbiol. 2007 Mar;73(6):2033–5.

59. Keita A, Brouqui P, Badiaga S, Benkouiten S, Ratmanov P, Raoult D, et al. *Tropheryma whipplei* prevalence strongly suggests human transmission in homeless shelters. Int J Infect Dis. 2013 Jan;17(1):e67–8.

60. Fenollar F, Keita A, Buffet S, Raoult D. Intrafamilial circulation of tropheryma whipplei. France Emerg Infect Dis. 2012;18(6):949–55.

61. Hujoel I, Johnson D, Lebwohl B, Leffler D, Kupfer S, Tsung-Teh W, et al. *Tropheryma whipplei* infection (Whipple disease) in the United States. Dig Dis Sci. 2019;64(1):213–23.

62. Schneider T, Moos V, Loddenkemper C, Marth T, Fenollar F, Raoult D. Whipple's disease: new aspects of pathogenesis and treatment. Lancet Infect Dis. 2008;8(3):179–90.

63. Fenollar F, Puechal X, Raoult D. Whipple's disease. N Engl J Med. 2007;356(1):55–66.

64. Sakai E, Higurashi T, Ohkubo H, Hosono K, Ueda A, Matsuhashi N, et al. Investigation of small bowel abnormalities in HIV-infected patients using capsule endoscopy. Gastroenterol Res Pract. 2017;2017:1932647.

65. Epple H, Allers K, Troger H, Kuhl A, Erben U, Fromm M, et al. Acute HIV infection induces mucosal infiltration with CD4+ and CD8+ T cells, epithelial apoptosis, and a mucosal barrier defect. Gastroenterology. 2010;139(4):1289–300.

66. Guadalupe M, Reay E, Sankaran S, Prindiville T, Flamm J, McNeil A, et al. Severe CD4+ T-cell depletion in gut lymphoid tissue during primary human immunodeficiency virus type 1 infection and substantial delay in restoration following highly active antiretroviral therapy. J Virol. 2003;77(21):11708–17.

67. Wang H, Kotler D. HIV enteropathy and aging: gastrointestinal immunity, mucosal epithelial barrier, and microbial translocation. Curr Opin HIV AIDS. 2014;9(4):309–16.

68. Greenson J, Belitsos P, Yardley J, Bartlett J. AIDS enteropathy: occult enteric infections and duodenal mucosal alterations in chronic diarrhea. Ann Intern Med. 1991;114(5):366–72.

69. Utay N, Somasunderam A, Hinkle J, Petschow B, Detzel C, Somsouk M, et al. Serum bovine immunoglobins improve inflammation and gut barrier function in persons with HIV and enteropathy on suppressive ART. Pathog Immun. 2019;4(1):124–46.

70. Troseid M, Manner I, Pedersen K, Haissman J, Kvale D, Nielsen S. Microbial translocation and cardiometabolic risk factors in HIV infection. AIDS Res Hum Retrovir. 2014;30(6):514–22.

71. Pipaliya N, Ingle M, Rathi C, Poddar P, Pandav N, Sawant P. Spectrum of chronic small bowel diarrhea with malabsorption in Indian subcontinent: is the trend really changing? Intest Res. 2016;14(1):75–82.

72. McCarroll M, Riddle M, Gutierrez R, Porter C. Infectious gastroenteritis as a risk factor for tropical sprue and malabsorption: a case-control study. Dig Dis Sci. 2015;60(11):3379–85.

73. Langenberg M, Wismans P, van Genderen P. Distinguishing tropical sprue from celiac disease in returning travellers with chronic diarrhoea: a diagnostic challenge? Travel Med Infect Dis. 2014;12(4):401–5.

74. Nath S. Tropical sprue. Curr Gastroenterol Rep. 2005;7:343–9.

75. Jacobs C, Coss Adame E, Attaluri A, Valestin J, Rao S. Dysmotility and proton pump inhibitor use are independent risk factors for small intestinal bacterial and/or fungal overgrowth. Aliment Pharmacol Ther. 2013;37(11):1103–11.

76. Choung R, Ruff K, Malhotra A, Herrick L, Locke GR, Harmsen W, et al. clinical predictors of small intestinal bacterial overgrowth by duodenal aspirate culture. Aliment Pharmacol Ther. 2011;33(9):1059–67.

77. Lasa J, Zubiaurre I, Fanjul I, Olivera P, Soifer L. Small intestinal bacterial overgrowth prevalence in celiac disease patients is similar in healthy subjects and lower in irritable bowel syndrome patients. Revista de Gastroenterologia de Mexico. 2015;80(2):171–4.

78. Lappinga P, Abraham S, Murray J, Vetter E, Patel R, Wu T. Small intestinal bacterial overgrowth: histopathologic features and clinical correlates in an underrecognized entity. Arch Pathol Lab Med. 2010;134(2):264–170.

79. Erdogan A, Rao S, Gulley D, Jacobs C, Lee Y, Badger C. Small intestinal bacterial overgrowth: duodenal aspiration vs glucose breath test. Neurogastroenterol Motil. 2015;27(4):481–9.

80. Ghoshal U, Ghoshal U. Small intestinal bacterial overgrowth and other intestinal disorders. Gastroenterol Clin N Am. 2017;46(1):103–20.

81. Rezaie A, Buresi M, Lembo A, Lin H, McCallum R, Rao S, et al. Hydrogen and methane-based breath testing in gastrointestinal disorders: the North American consensus. Am J Gastroenterol. 2017;112(5):775–84.

82. Gatta L, Scarpignato C. Systematic review with meta-analysis: rifaximin is effective and safe for the treatment of small intestine bacterial overgrowth. Aliment Pharmacol Ther. 2017;45:604–16.

83. Zhong C, Qu C, Wang B, Liang S, Zeng B. Probiotics for preventing and treating small intestinal bacterial overgrowth: a meta-analysis and systematic review of current evidence. J Clin Gastroenterol. 2017;51(4):300–11.

84. Vakiani E, Arguelles-Grande C, Mansukhani M, Lewis S, Rotterdamn H, Green P, et al. Collagenous sprue is not always associated with dismal outcomes: a clinicopathological study of 19 patients. Mod Pathol. 2010;23(1):12–26.

85. Nielsen J, Steephen A, Lewin M. Angiotensin-II inhibitor (olmesartan)-induced collagenosu sprue with resolution following discontinuation of drug. World J Gastroenterol. 2013;19(40):6928–30.

86. Vasant D, Hayes S, Bucknall R, Lal S. Clinical and histological resolution fo collagenous sprue following gluten-free diet and discontinuation of non-steroidal anti-inflammatory drugs (NSAIDs). BMJ Case Rep. 2013;2013:bcr2013200097.

87. Rubio-Tapia A, Talley N, Gurudu S, Wu T, Murray J. Gluten-free diet and steroid treatment are effective therapy for most patients with collagenous sprue. Clin Gastroenterol Hepatol. 2010;8(4):344–9.

88. Freeman H. Hyposplenism, antiendomysial antibodies and lymphocytic colitis in collagenous sprue. Can J Gastroenterol. 1999;13(4):347–50.

89. Maguire A, Greenson J, Lauwers G, Ginsburg R, Williams G, Brown I, et al. Collagenous sprue: a clinicopathologic study of 12 cases. Am J Surg Pathol. 2009;33(10):1440–9.

90. Robert M, Ament M, Weinstein W. The histologic spectrum and clinical outcome of refractory and unclassified sprue. Am J Surg Pathol. 2000;24(5):676–87.
91. Schmidt C, Kasim E, Schlake W, Gerken G, Giese T, Stallmach A. TNF-alpha antibody treatment in refractory collagenous sprue: report of a case and review of the literature. Z Gastroenterol. 2009;47(6):575–8.
92. Jensen E, Martin C, Kappelman M, Dellon E. Prevalence of eosinophilic gastritis, gastroenteritis, and colitis: estimates from a national administrative database. J Pediatr Gastroenterol Nutr. 2016;62(1):36–42.
93. Spergel J, Book W, Mays E, Song L, Shah S, Talley N, et al. Variation in prevalence, diagnostic criteria, and initial management options for eosinophilic gastrointestinal diseases in the United States. J Pediatr Gastroenterol Nutr. 2011;52(3):300–6.
94. Talley N, Shorter R, Phillips S, Zinsmeister A. Eosinophilic gastroenteritis: a clinicopathological study of patients with disease of the mucosa, muscle layer, and subserosal tissues. Gut. 1990;31(1):54–8.
95. Klein N, Hargrove R, Sleisenger M, Jeffries G. Eosinophilic gastroenteritis. Medicine (Baltimore). 1970;49(4):299–319.
96. Chang J, Choung R, Lee R, Locke GR, Schleck C, Zinsmeister A, et al. A shift in the clinical spectrum of eosinophliic gastroenteritis toward the mucosal disease type. Clin Gastroenterol Hepatol. 2010;8(8):669–75.
97. Reed C, Woosley J, Dellon E. Clinical characteristics, treatment outcomes, and resource utilization in children and adults with eosinophilic gastroenteritis. Dig Liver Dis. 2015;47(3):197–201.
98. Butterfield J, Murray J. Eosinophilic gastroenteritis and gluten-sensitive enteropathy in the same patient. J Clin Gastroenterol. 2002;34(5):552–3.
99. Tien F, Wu J, Jeng Y, Hsu H, Ni Y, Chang M, et al. Clinical features and treatment responses of children with eosinophilic gastroenteritis. Pediatr Neonatol. 2011;52(5):272–8.
100. Zheng X, Cheng J, Pan K, Yang K, Wang H, Wu E. Eosinophilic enteritis: CT features. Abdom Imaging. 2008;33(2):191–5.
101. Wong G, Lim K, Wan W, Low S, Kong S. Eosinophilic gastroenteritis: clinical profiles and treatment outcomes, a retrospective study of 18 adult patients in a Singapore tertiary hospital. Med J Malaysia. 2015;70(4):232–7.
102. Hurrell J, Genta R, Melton S. Histopathologic diagnosis of eosinophilic conditions in the gastrointestinal tract. Adv Anat Pathol. 2011;18(5):335–48.
103. Pineton de Chambrun G, Gonzalez F, Canva J, Gonzalez S, Houssin L, Desremaux P, et al. Natural history of eosinophilic gastroenteritis. Clin Gastroenterol Hepatol. 2011;9(11):950–6.

# Treatment of Refractory Celiac Disease

G. Bouma and T. Dieckman

## Introduction

A small subset of celiac disease (CD) patients is, or becomes, refractory to a gluten-free diet with persistent malabsorption and intestinal villous atrophy. The most common cause of this condition is inadvertent gluten exposure but concomitant diseases and alternative diagnoses resulting in villous atrophy should also be considered and excluded. Patients are referred to as refractory celiac disease when these causes are excluded. Two types are recognized, based on the absence (RCD type I) or presence (RCD type II) of a clonal expansion of premalignant intra-epithelial lymphocyte (IEL) population with a high potential for transformation into an overt enteropathy-associated T-cell lymphoma (EATL). The definition, epidemiology, pathogenesis and diagnostic armamentarium of RCD have been described in detail in previous Chapters. Here, we will focus on the pharmacological approaches that have been evaluated so far for both types of RCD.

When evaluating treatment outcomes it is important to bear in mind several considerations.

First, the definition of refractory celiac disease. It is now generally accepted that the definition for type 2 disease is based on the percentage and immunophenotype of a subset of IELs with an abnormal or 'aberrant' phenotype as determined by flow cytometry [1]. Earlier diagnostic approaches, including immunohistochemistry and TCR clonality analysis had lower sensitivities and specificities [2]. Consequently, patients categorized as type 2 patients might have been classified as type 1 and *vice versa* according to the diagnostic approach and definition. For type 1 disease no such gold standard exists. In fact, a significant proportion of patients with inadvertent gluten consumption, a slow histological response to the gluten free diet or a

G. Bouma (✉) · T. Dieckman
Celiac Disease Center, Department of Gastroenterology and Hepatology, Amsterdam University Medical Center, Research Institute AGEM, Amsterdam, the Netherlands
e-mail: g.bouma@amsterdamumc.nl; t.dieckman@amsterdamumc.nl

© Springer Nature Switzerland AG 2022
G. Malamut, N. Cerf-Bensussan (eds.), *Refractory Celiac Disease*,
https://doi.org/10.1007/978-3-030-90142-4_9

concomitant disease such as microscopic colitis may have erroneously been classified as having refractory disease. In this regard, the duration of the gluten free diet is particularly relevant. Some authors adhere to a 6 months period since the start of the gluten free diet, others to 12 months. Yet, it should be noted that histologic recovery, especially in elderly patients may be substantially longer [3, 4].

Second, in RCD type 2, there is marked heterogeneity in the intra-epithelial lymphocyte (IEL) compartment. Previous work from Schmitz et al. has shown two major aberrant IEL populations in RCDII patients: CD56−CD127− and CD56−CD127+ [5]. Experiments evaluating the intestinal innate IEL compartment of non-CD patients as well as CD patients, revealed that the IL-2/-15 receptor B chain (CD122) is expressed by the lineage-negative CD56−CD127− population in contrast to the CD56−CD127+ population which showed lower expression of CD122. In contrast, the latter population showed co-expression of the IL-21 receptor and IL-15 receptor α-chain. What also stresses heterogeneity is the observation that the clonality of T-cell receptor rearrangements differed between RCDII cell lines as well as within a relatively large group of RCDII patients [6]. Furthermore, aberrant IELs display different stages of maturity between RCDII patients, of which only the patients harbouring the most mature aberrant IEL population developed an EATL [6]. Besides these diverse inter-individual differences, aberrant IELs in RCDII might also be characterized by intra-individual heterogeneity as RCDII cell lines show fractioned expression of different γ-chain receptors within one cell line [5]. More recent unpublished work using mass cytometry of individual celiac patients has confirmed and further defined the marked heterogeneity of the aberrant IEL population in RCDII.

A third point to consider is that both forms of RCD are extremely rare. This has precluded, with so far one exception, placebo-controlled clinical trials. Virtually all data come from case reports or uncontrolled small case series with established anti-inflammatory or immunomodulatory drugs used in other immune-mediated diseases, on a trial and error base. Finally, in particular in type 2 disease, there are no predefined endpoints. Different studies have used different outcome measures, including clinical improvement, restoration of villous architecture, reduction in aberrant cells and prevention of EATL.

In the next section we will discuss the published studies and discuss the evidence for the various drugs investigated so far in light of the above mentioned considerations.

## Overview of the Drugs Investigated in Refractory Celiac Disease

The first descriptions of refractory celiac disease date back to the late seventies of the last century with the description of a 63 year old male with recurrence of malabsorption and villous atrophy 5 years after diagnosis and successful treatment of celiac disease. Treatment with corticosteroids resulted in partial recovery of villous architecture yet he remained steroid dependent [7]. At that time also the first cases of non-responsive CeD treated with thiopurines were described [8, 9].

In the early nineties a case report described remission of severe sprue after receiving cyclosporine therapy in a patient who was unresponsive to a gluten-free diet and corticosteroid therapy [10]. Shortly thereafter a similar effect of azathioprine was described in a patient with nongranulomatous ulcerative jejunoileitis [11].

At that time there was no concept of the etiopathogenesis of refractory sprue. The suggestion that patients with refractory disease can progress to an overt T cell lymphoma and that refractory celiac disease is in fact a cryptic T-cell lymphoma was first suggested by Carbonnel et al in 1998 [12]. In the same year Cellier et al. demonstrated that refractory sprue is associated with an abnormal subset of intraepithelial lymphocytes containing CD3 epsilon but lacking surface expression of T-cell receptors and restricted rearrangements of the T cell receptor gamma chain [13]. Shortly thereafter it was shown that in ulcerative jejunitis and refractory celiac disease the monoclonal T-cell population is constituted by cytologically normal, noninvasive intraepithelial T lymphocytes that share an identical aberrant immunophenotype with EATL [14]. These observations and the ongoing research in understanding the etiopathogenesis of RCD have paved the way for novel therapeutic approaches that are currently underway.

## Immunosuppressive and Immunomodulatory Drugs

### Systemic Corticosteroids and Budesonide

Systemic corticosteroids have been widely used in both type 1 and 2 patients, both alone and in conjunction with other immune modulating therapies, yet there are no studies that have specifically studied effectiveness. The picture that emerges from these observations is that steroids are clinically effective to induce clinical remission and mucosal recovery in most patients with RCD type 1 (for a review: see [15]). Clinical response to steroids is also observed in the majority (~75%) of patients with RCD type 2, however mucosal recovery is infrequent and progression to EATL is not prevented [16–18].

The use of budesonide has been evaluated in three studies. The first was a series of nine patients [19], including four with RCD type I and three with RCD type II with signs of early T cell lymphoma. Treatment with Entocort™ was clinically effective in all four with RCD type I but not in two out of three RCD type 2 patients. Another case series evaluated 29 patients, including five patients with type II disease based on the presence of a clonal T-cell population. Five patients were on a gluten free diet for less than 6 months, 31% had persistent positive antibodies and seven had concomitant microscopic colitis. Definition of response was based on symptoms and number of daily bowel movements. Overall, 76% of patients responded to the medication, 55% completely when used alone or with oral corticosteroids and/or azathioprine. Of five RCD type 2 patients, four had improvement of symptoms, not otherwise specified. While there was an objective improvement in the number of bowel movements in those who responded, there was no improvement in the duodenal biopsy over the study period for a mean of 6.7 ± 8.5 months [20].

The largest study that has evaluated the effect of budesonide included 57 patients who received open capsule budesonide for suspected RCD [21]. Based on clonal T-cell receptor gamma gene rearrangement or aberrant phenotype of intraepithelial lymphocytes (IELs), 13 patients (23%) were classified as having RCD-2 and 43 (75%) as RCD-1. Prior immunomodulating treatment including azathioprine, systemic corticosteroids, or regular budesonide had failed in nearly half. Following therapy for a median of 22 months, the majority had clinical (92%) and histologic (89%) improvement. Follow-up biopsy in seven out of 13 patients with RCD-2 (53%) showed an absence of clonal TCR gamma gene rearrangement or aberrant IEL phenotype previously seen. On follow-up, two patients (4%) died of enteropathy-associated T-cell lymphoma.

## Cyclosporin

After the initial case reports on cyclosporine, a case series of 13 patients was published in 2000 [22]. Refractory CD in this study was defined as malabsorption in the presence of gluten-related partial, subtotal or total villous atrophy in the small intestinal biopsy in patients with established CD on a gluten free diet for at least 1 year. After the 2-month treatment period histological improvement was seen in six patients. Continuation of cyclosporin medication resulted in (further) improvement of histology in three patients. Overall, in eight of the 13 patients in the study group improvement of small intestinal histology was seen. Normalization of villi, i.e. recovery to Marsh I–II was seen in five of these eight patients (38% of the study group). Despite these initial positive results there have been no follow-up studies to substantiate these observations.

## Thiopurines

Following the first case reports on the effectiveness of Azathioprine, a prospective open label study from 2002 evaluated Azathioprine in seven patients for a mean of 11 months (range 8–12 months) [23]. Patients had a well-defined diagnosis of refractory sprue and a lack of response to oral or parenteral steroids. Five patients had endoscopic evidence of ulcerative jejunitis, and monoclonal TCR gamma gene rearrangement was shown in five of six patients studied, suggestive of RCD type 2. Two patients had persistent positive anti-endomysial and anti-tTG antibodies. Following treatment, five patients had a complete clinical remission, and biochemical and nutritional parameters were significantly improved. Steroids were tapered after the onset of azathioprine, and no patient was on steroids at the end of the study.

Intestinal histology improved significantly in all cases (normal histology in three cases and minor infiltration in the lamina propria in two). Two patients did not respond to treatment and died due to unrelated causes, and a third one during follow-up. No overt lymphoma was demonstrated during follow-up. Despite the high mortality seen in this group of patients it was concluded that azathioprine might be a valid and effective drug for the treatment of RCD. Similarly, a single case report [24] also demonstrated clinical and histological normalization after institution of azathioprine in a refractory patient. No information was available for this patient on the percentage of aberrant cells or T cell clonality.

This tentative optimism was contrasted by the finding that in a series of eight patients with refractory celiac type 2 (i.e., with confirmed increased numbers of lymphocytes with an aberrant phenotype), six developed an overt enteropathy associated T cell lymphoma [25]. In the same study, improvement of small intestinal histology with a decrease of intra-epithelial lymphocytosis was seen in eight of ten RCD type I patients with restoration of normal villous architecture in four.

Another retrospective observational study [26] analyzed the effectiveness of tioguanine, a thiopurine related to azathioprine which requires less metabolic conversion towards the active metabolite. Twelve adult refractory coeliac disease type I patients with a median TG treatment duration of 14 months and a follow-up of at least 1 year were included. Clinical and histological response rates were 83% and 78%, respectively whereas corticosteroid dependency decreased by 50%. Two patients withdrew treatment due to adverse events. No liver related side effects were seen in any of the patients.

## IL-10

Interleukin-10 (IL-10) is a cytokine with potent anti-inflammatory and immuno-regulatory functions. The effectiveness of rHu IL-10 was studied in a series of 10 patients with refractory CD [27]. Refractoriness was defined as recurrent malabsorption in the presence of villous atrophy in the small intestinal mucosa in patients with strict adherence to a GFD for at least 3 years and low or stable anti-gliadin antibodies (<100 U/l) for at least 2 months. IL-10, given during a 3 month period dosage was not overall effective; two patients had to discontinue treatment because of side effects. The primary endpoint, i.e., normalization of villous architecture was seen in only one patient with another patient showing improvement of abnormalities.

## Anti-TNF

Infliximab was given to a 47 year old patient with refractory celiac disease unresponsive to steroids and partially responsive to cyclosporin [28]. Whether or not this case reflects a type 2 refractory patient is unknown, but appears less likely as there was no evidence for T-cell receptor gene rearrangement. A single infusion of

Infliximab dramatically improved symptoms and patient could be weaned off steroids and duodenal mucosa returned to normality with a normal villous architecture after which she was switched to azathioprine. Follow-up during 18 months showed persistent remission both clinically and histologically. Similarly, in another case of refractory coeliac disease not otherwise specified [29], remission was induced by a single infusion of infliximab and was maintained with prednisolone and azathioprine for 1 year. It should be noted that refractoriness in this case was not confirmed by normalization of serology.

Finally a 14-year-old girl with persistent symptoms and positive tissue celiac-specific antibodies despite a gluten-free diet was treated with infliximab with subsequent complete serological and histological remission [30].

## Mesalamine

One study evaluated mesalamine for symptom relief in refractory celiac disease (RCD) [31]. Refractoriness was defined as persisting clinical and histological abnormalities in patients who were strictly adherent to the gluten-free diet for at least 6 months. Based on immunohistochemical findings patients were classified as type 1 patients. Four patients were treated with a special formulation for proximal release of mesalamine (Small intestinal release mesalamine; SIRM) and six received SIRM and oral budesonide. Within 4 weeks, 50% had complete response and an additional 10% had partial symptom response. Two of the six patients were able to discontinue budesonide.

## *Cytoreductive Drugs*

The realization that RCD type 2 is in fact a low grade lymphoma and emerging insight in the mechanisms by which these cells exert tissue damage has led to strategies to specifically target the aberrant cells and the cytotoxic mediators they secrete.

## Alemtuzumab

Alemtuzumab, a monoclonal antibody against CD52 used in cases of chronic lymphocytic leukemia was administered to a single patient with refractory celiac disease type 2 for 12 consecutive weeks [32]. After 9 months of treatment, the patient remained asymptomatic. Prednisone was withdrawn after 8 weeks of alemtuzumab therapy with total recovery of villous architecture. In another patient clinical symptoms improved, yet villous atrophy persisted, and the percentage of aberrant intraepithelial increased while on treatment [33].

## Cladribine

Cladribine (2-CDA) is a synthetic purine analogue that causes cell death by accumulation of cytotoxic cladribine triphosphates in cells with high expression of the enzyme deoxycytidine kinase, including T cells. The rationale for the use in RCD was based on the effectiveness of this drug in hairy cell leukemia, a disease also characterized by CD103 positive pathologic cells. In a series of 17 patients (eight men, nine women) with established RCD2 Cladribine was given for one to three cycles [34]. Six patients (35.8%) showed a clinical improvement (*i.e.,* weight gain, improvement of diarrhea, and hypoalbuminemia). In 10 patients (58.8%) a significant histologic improvement was seen, including the disappearance of ulcerative jejunitis lesions in all five patients. In six patients (35.2%) a significant decrease in aberrant T cells was seen. Nevertheless, seven patients (41.1%) developed EATL and died subsequently, three of them within 7 months after Cladribine treatment.

As an extension of this study, a retrospective analysis of RCD II patients treated with 2-CdA was performed in 32 patients (including 14 patients from the previous study) with a median follow-up of 31 months [35]. Clinical course, histological and immunological response rates as well as survival rate, and occurrence of enteropathy associated T-cell lymphoma (EATL) were evaluated. Overall, 18 patients responded to 2-CdA, of which 7 (22%) had both clinical, histological and immunological responses. Those who did responded had a statistically significant increased survival compared to those who were unresponsive; overall 3- and 5-year survival was 83% in those who clinically responded to Cladribine therapy versus 63% and 22% in the non-responder group. Overall, 12 patients (37%) died, of which five due to progression to EATL. Notably, among the different response parameters, the presence or absence of a histological response rather than decrease in the number of aberrant cells [36], was predictive for EATL development in patients treated with Cladribine and may be instrumental in the decision to a more aggressive treatment with autologous stem cell transplantation.

## Stem Cell Transplantation

A potential more definitive solution for refractory celiac disease is to induce immunoablation with high dose chemotherapy followed by regeneration of naive T lymphocytes derived from reinfused autologous hematopoietic progenitor cells. This approach has been applied in several autoimmune diseases and initial analysis of seven RCD II patients demonstrated that this approach is feasible and well tolerated in type 2 refractory celiac patients [37]. There was a significant reduction in the aberrant T cells in duodenal biopsies associated with improvement in clinical well-being and normalization of hematologic and biochemical markers after a mean follow-up of 15.5 months; range, 7–30 months). One patient died 8 months after transplantation from progressive neuroceliac disease. As an extension of this initial observation, 18 RCD II patients were evaluated for auto-SCT [38]. Five patients could not be transplanted and all died. Thirteen patients were transplanted successfully and followed for >2 years. One patient died of EATL in this group. The most recent report on this patient cohort included 15 transplanted patients with a median follow-up of 78 months (range: 18–196 months). One patient developed EATL; 1- and 5-year survival rates were 100% and 85% respectively.

Together, these data demonstrate that 2-CDA-auSCT step-up therapy and 2-CdA monotherapy show a good and comparable effect on EATL prevention and overall survival in those patients who achieve histological remission. Patients who fail to respond histologically on 2-CDA monotherapy are at risk for EATL development and should be considered for an additional step-up strategy consisting of auto-SCT and/or newly developed treatment regimens.

## Mesenchymal Stem Cell Transplantation

Another therapeutic approach that may be beneficial in RCD patients takes advantage of the regenerative and immunomodulatory properties of mesenchymal stem cells (MSCs). So far there is one case report of a woman with RCD type 2 who underwent repeated infusions of autologous mesenchymal stem cells [39]. There were no adverse effects and a profound effect on her clinical condition was seen, including normalization of mucosal architecture. Nevertheless the aberrant IEL population persisted, similar to the observations after autologous stem cell transplantation. A possible explanation may relate to the inhibitory effects on proliferation of IL-15–stimulated cells by mesenchymal stem cells [40]. Indeed, in this patient it was observed that expression of IL-15 and its receptor almost completely disappeared after MSC treatment.

### Novel Approaches

The chronic upregulation of IL-15 in the epithelium and in the intestinal lamina propria (LP) is a hallmark of celiac disease and correlates with the degree of mucosal damage. In the case of RCDII, sustained expression of high levels of IL-15 in the epithelium leads to the expansion of the aberrant cell population. Additionally, IL-15 has an anti-apoptotic effect on aberrant IELs and finally somatic JAK1 or STAT3 gain-of-function mutations (or both) confer hyper-responsiveness to IL-15 which further augments the massive expansion of this cell population. In ex-vivo cultures of intestinal biopsies from patients with RCDII, neutralization of IL-15 using monoclonal antibodies blocked anti-apoptotic signaling via JAK3 and STAT5 and led to apoptosis of the clonal aberrant IEL's. These findings lend support to the potential clinical effectiveness of IL-15 blockade. To address this question, celiac disease patients on a gluten free diet underwent a gluten challenge in conjunction with either placebo or AMG 714 [41], a fully human immunoglobulin monoclonal antibody (IgG1κ) that binds to IL-15 and inhibits IL-15-induced T-cell activation and proliferation. While clinical symptoms were ameliorated with AMG 714 treatment between baseline and week 12, treatment did not prevent mucosal injury due to gluten challenge. In a parallel randomized study in 28 patients with RCD type 2, treatment for 12 week did show some effect on clinical symptoms but again did not result in significant changes in histology or percentage of aberrant cells when treated patients were compared with placebo treated controls [42].

# Conclusion

## Looking Back and Looking Forward: Future Perspectives on Treatment of Refractory Celiac Disease

Almost five decades have passed since the first case description of refractory celiac disease. Two distinct manifestations of refractory celiac disease are recognized; RCDI, the benign form, and the potentially malignant form RCDII characterized by clonal expansion of aberrant IELs. Clear diagnostic criteria for refractory celiac disease type 2 have been defined but novel molecular and genetic markers will further refine the heterogeneity of type 2 disease.

For type 1 disease there is currently no gold standard and diagnosis is largely *per exclusionem*. This also hampers comparison of different treatments. The picture that has emerged from studies so far is that disease has a benign course and benefits from various regimens including immunosuppressive and immunomodulatory drugs like (topical) steroids, thiopurines and anti-TNF. Open-capsule budesonide has been proposed as a standard first-line therapy for both type I and type II refractory celiac disease, as long as the latter is stable. Refractory celiac disease falls under the umbrella classification of "slow responders". In the absence of controlled studies it cannot be excluded at this point that in a proportion of patients a wait-and-see policy would have yielded comparable results and prospective studies that address this question are urgently needed.

As for type 2 disease, pre-defined end points are needed to compare the different therapeutic options. Apart from anti-IL15, there are no controlled studies and all rely on case reports or small (retrospective) case series which precludes firm conclusions. IL-10 can definitely be disregarded as treatment option and as far as thiopurines, there is at least concern that it may promote progression to overt lymphoma. The observation that a patient with RCDII who received fecal microbiota transfer as treatment for a recurrent Clostridium difficile infection showed a full recovery of duodenal villi warrants further exploration [43].

Cyclosporin has shown beneficial effects in a small series of patients but this requires confirmation in an independent data set. The same accounts for budesonide. Data on Cladribine treatment show clinical effectiveness but appears not to prevent progression to EATL. Interestingly, mucosal recovery rather than reduction in the number of aberrant cells appears to be associated with a low risk to progress to EATL and this may be an important future outcome parameter. In those who do not respond histologically, autologous stem cell transplantation may be effective in risk reduction for the development of EATL. Monotherapy of anti-IL-15 appears not sufficient to interfere with the inflammatory cascade in RCD and the marked heterogeneity of the aberrant IEL cell compartment may contribute to the lack of overall effectiveness. Indeed, recent data show that IL-15 is up-regulated in only a subset of CD patients [44, 45]. In addition, a sizeable subset of malignant Lin⁻IELs in RCDII patients express low amounts of CD122, suggesting poor IL-15 responsiveness [5]. The observation that TNF, IL-2, and IL-21 as CD4⁺ T-cell cytokines act synergistically with IL-15 on survival and expansion of the malignant Lin⁻IEL population suggest that drugs that more broadly target cytokine signaling may be an attractive alternative strategy to counter the expansion of malignant Lin⁻IELs in RCDII patients [46]. Since these cytokines all mediate their intracellular effects through JAK-STAT signaling, and there is hyperresponsive of aberrant cells by JAK1/STAT3 mutations [47, 48], blockade of this pathway by Tofacitinib, an oral JAK1/JAK3 inhibitor is a logical candidate and currently investigated in a Phase 2 trial (clinicaltrialsregister.eu, NTR 7529; EudraCT 2018-001678-10).

# References

1. van Wanrooij RLJ, et al. Accurate classification of RCD requires flow cytometry. Gut. 2010;59(12):1732.
2. van Wanrooij RLJ, et al. Optimal strategies to identify aberrant intra-epithelial lymphocytes in refractory coeliac disease. J Clin Immunol. 2014;34(7):828–35.
3. Lanzini A, et al. Complete recovery of intestinal mucosa occurs very rarely in adult coeliac patients despite adherence to gluten-free diet. Aliment Pharmacol Ther. 2009;29(12):1299–308.
4. Wahab PJ, Meijer JWR, Mulder CJJ. Histologic follow-up of people with celiac disease on a gluten-free diet: slow and incomplete recovery. Am J Clin Pathol. 2002;118(3):459–63.
5. Schmitz F, et al. Identification of a potential physiological precursor of aberrant cells in refractory coeliac disease type II. Gut. 2013;62(4):509.
6. Tack GJ, et al. Origin and immunophenotype of aberrant IEL in RCDII patients. Mol Immunol. 2012;50(4):262–70.
7. Trier JS, et al. Celiac sprue and refractory sprue. Gastroenterology. 1978;75(2):307–16.
8. Hillman HS. Intestinal malabsorption with subtotal villous atrophy unresponsive to a gluten-free diet but responding to immunosuppressive therapy. Med J Aust. 1972;2(2):82–4.
9. Hamilton JD, Chambers RA, Wynn-Williams A. Role of gluten, prednisone, and azathioprine in non-responsive coeliac disease. Lancet. 1976;1(7971):1213–6.
10. Longstreth GF. Successful treatment of refractory sprue with cyclosporine. Ann Intern Med. 1993;119(10):1014–6.
11. Enns R, Lay T, Bridges R. Use of axathioprine for nongranulomatous ulcerative jejunoileitis. Can J Gastroenterol. 1997;11:589581.
12. Carbonnel F, et al. Are complicated forms of celiac disease cryptic T-cell lymphomas? Blood. 1998;92(10):3879–86.
13. Cellier C, et al. Abnormal intestinal intraepithelial lymphocytes in refractory sprue. Gastroenterology. 1998;114(3):471–81.
14. Bagdi E, et al. Mucosal intra-epithelial lymphocytes in enteropathy-associated T-cell lymphoma, ulcerative jejunitis, and refractory celiac disease constitute a neoplastic population. Blood. 1999;94(1):260–4.

15. Rubio-Tapia A, Murray JA. Classification and management of refractory coeliac disease. Gut. 2010;59(4):547.
16. Al-Toma A, et al. Survival in refractory coeliac disease and enteropathy-associated T-cell lymphoma: retrospective evaluation of single-centre experience. Gut. 2007;56(10):1373–8.
17. Malamut G, et al. Presentation and long-term follow-up of refractory celiac disease: comparison of type I with type II. Gastroenterology. 2009;136(1):81–90.
18. Rubio–Tapia A, et al. Clinical staging and survival in refractory celiac disease: a single center experience. Gastroenterology. 2009;136(1):99–107.
19. Daum S, et al. Therapy with budesonide in patients with refractory sprue. Digestion. 2006;73(1):60–8.
20. Brar P, et al. Budesonide in the treatment of refractory celiac disease. Am J Gastroenterol. 2007;102(10):2265–9.
21. Mukewar SS, et al. Open-capsule budesonide for refractory celiac disease. Am J Gastroenterol. 2017;112(6):959–67.
22. Wahab PJ, et al. Cyclosporin in the treatment of adults with refractory coeliac disease—an open pilot study. Aliment Pharmacol Ther. 2000;14(6):767–74.
23. Mauriño E, et al. Azathioprine in refractory sprue: results from a prospective, open-label study. Am J Gastroenterol. 2002;97(10):2595–602.
24. Iqbal U, et al. Refractory celiac disease successfully treated with azathioprine. Gastroenterology Res. 2017;10(3):199–201.
25. Goerres MS, et al. Azathioprine and prednisone combination therapy in refractory coeliac disease. Aliment Pharmacol Ther. 2003;18(5):487–94.
26. Tack GJ, et al. Tioguanine in the treatment of refractory coeliac disease - a single centre experience. Aliment Pharmacol Ther. 2012;36(3):274–81.
27. Mulder C, Wahab PJ, Meijer JW, Metselaar E. A pilot study of recombinant human interleukin-10 in adults with refractory coeliac disease. Eur J Gastroenterol Hepatol. 2001;13(10):1183–8.
28. Gillett HR, et al. Successful infliximab treatment for steroid-refractory celiac disease: a case report. Gastroenterology. 2002;122(3):800–5.
29. Turner SM, Moorghen M, Probert CS. Refractory coeliac disease: remission with infliximab and immunomodulators. Eur J Gastroenterol Hepatol. 2005;17(6):667–9.
30. Rawal N, et al. Remission of refractory celiac disease with infliximab in a pediatric patient. ACG Case Rep J. 2015;2(2):121–3.
31. Jamma S, et al. Small intestinal release mesalamine for the treatment of refractory celiac disease type I. J Clin Gastroenterol. 2011;45(1):30–3.
32. Vivas S, et al. Alemtuzumab for refractory celiac disease in a patient at risk for enteropathy-associated T-cell lymphoma. N Engl J Med. 2006;354(23):2514–5.
33. Verbeek WH, Mulder C, Zweegman S. Alemtuzumab for refractory celiac disease. N Engl J Med. 2006;355(13):1396–7.
34. Al-Toma A, et al. Cladribine therapy in refractory celiac disease with aberrant T cells. Clin Gastroenterol Hepatol. 2006;4(11):1322–7. quiz 1300
35. Tack GJ, et al. Evaluation of cladribine treatment in refractory celiac disease type II. World J Gastroenterol. 2011;17(4):506–13.
36. Nijeboer P, et al. Lymphoma development and survival in refractory coeliac disease type II: histological response as prognostic factor. United European Gastroenterol J. 2017;5(2):208–17.
37. Al-toma A, et al. Autologous hematopoietic stem cell transplantation in refractory celiac disease with aberrant T cells. Blood. 2006;109(5):2243–9.
38. Tack GJ, et al. Auto-SCT in refractory celiac disease type II patients unresponsive to cladribine therapy. Bone Marrow Transplant. 2011;46(6):840–6.
39. Ciccocioppo R, et al. A refractory celiac patient successfully treated with mesenchymal stem cell infusions. Mayo Clin Proc. 2016;91(6):812–9.

40. Spaggiari GM, et al. Mesenchymal stem cells inhibit natural killer–cell proliferation, cytotoxicity, and cytokine production: role of indoleamine 2,3-dioxygenase and prostaglandin E2. Blood. 2008;111(3):1327–33.
41. Lähdeaho ML, et al. Safety and efficacy of AMG 714 in adults with coeliac disease exposed to gluten challenge: a phase 2a, randomised, double-blind, placebo-controlled study. Lancet Gastroenterol Hepatol. 2019;4(12):948–59.
42. Cellier C, et al. Safety and efficacy of AMG 714 in patients with type 2 refractory coeliac disease: a phase 2a, randomised, double-blind, placebo-controlled, parallel-group study. Lancet Gastroenterol Hepatol. 2019;4(12):960–70.
43. van Beurden YH, et al. Serendipity in refractory celiac disease: full recovery of duodenal villi and clinical symptoms after fecal microbiota transfer. J Gastrointestin Liver Dis. 2016;25(3):385–8.
44. Bernardo D, et al. Higher constitutive IL15R alpha expression and lower IL-15 response threshold in coeliac disease patients. Clin Exp Immunol. 2008;154(1):64–73.
45. Abadie V, Jabri B. IL-15: a central regulator of celiac disease immunopathology. Immunol Rev. 2014;260(1):221–34.
46. Kooy-Winkelaar YM, et al. CD4 T-cell cytokines synergize to induce proliferation of malignant and nonmalignant innate intraepithelial lymphocytes. Proc Natl Acad Sci U S A. 2017;114(6):E980–9.
47. Soderquist CR, et al. Immunophenotypic spectrum and genomic landscape of refractory celiac disease type II. Am J Surg Pathol. 2021;45(7):905–16.
48. Cording S, et al. Oncogenetic landscape of lymphomagenesis in coeliac disease. bioRxiv. 2020; 2020.09.07.275032

# Prognosis of Refractory Coeliac Disease: The Prognostic Scores

Annalisa Schiepatti and Federico Biagi

## Introduction

Coeliac disease (CD) is a common chronic gluten-dependent enteropathy characterised by both a high prevalence in the general population [1, 2] and an increased morbidity and mortality, mostly due to refractory coeliac disease (RCD) and the other complications [3, 4]. Since most complications of CD are part of the same pathological spectrum and since they are almost indistinguishable from a clinical point of view, providing an overview on the prognosis of RCD cannot be separated from dealing with prognosis of complicated coeliac disease (CCD). Therefore, in this chapter we will first define the concept of complicated CD. Then, we will outline and discuss risk factors for developing RCD and CCD (i.e. predictors that can be evaluated at time of diagnosis of CD). Finally, we will deal with negative prognostic factors for RCD and CCD (i.e. factors that can be evaluated at time of diagnosis of complication). All these predictors may be useful in clinical practice to identify patients at higher risk of poor outcomes who may require a stricter follow-up and more aggressive and targeted therapies.

## Defining Complicated Coeliac Disease

Although the first papers introducing the concept of complications of CD were published more than 20 years ago [4–7], there is still no clear consensus on the definition of CCD [3–10]. In our opinion, it is crucial to distinguish between the true complications of CD, which are responsible for the increased mortality of coeliac patients, and conditions that are merely associated to CD and can be considered as

A. Schiepatti · F. Biagi (✉)

Gastroenterology Unit, IRCCS Pavia, ICS Maugeri, University of Pavia, Pavia, Italy

e-mail: annalisa.schiepatti01@universitadipavia.it; federico.biagi@icsmaugeri.it

© Springer Nature Switzerland AG 2022

G. Malamut, N. Cerf-Bensussan (eds.), *Refractory Celiac Disease*,

https://doi.org/10.1007/978-3-030-90142-4_10

part of the clinical presentation of CD itself. This group of associated conditions includes disorders such as osteoporosis [11, 12], persistent anaemia [13], autoimmune conditions [14, 15] and even obstetrical and gynaecological disorders [16]. These conditions have been considered by some authors among the complications of CD [10]. However, since it is debatable that they severely worsen the prognosis of coeliac patients, we would rather consider them as major long-term comorbidities associated to CD. In our opinion, true complications of CD are a group of abdominal pre-malignant and malignant conditions arising more frequently in coeliac patients than in the general population and well-known to be directly responsible for the increased mortality registered in coeliac patients [reviewed in 3]. These conditions are represented by RCD [17], ulcerative jejuno-ileitis (UJI) [18], enteropathy associated T-cell lymphoma (EATL) [19], abdominal B-cell lymphomas (ABL) [20], and small bowel carcinoma (SBC) [21]. Is it possible to consider them all together as CCD? Given their premalignant or malignant nature, their common origin from the abdomen, and a similar clinical picture characterised by severe symptoms of malabsorption (diarrhoea, weight loss, and anaemia), fever and abdominal pain, we think that the term complicated coeliac disease can be adopted to refer to these conditions as a whole [3, 4, 22–25]. Although these disorders are heterogeneous in terms of underlying molecular pathways [3, 4, 22–25], type 2 RCD and EATL may share pathogenetic mechanisms as suggested by the presence of the same aberrant intraepithelial lymphocyte (IELs) population [7]. These are the reasons why some of the papers addressing the issue of prognosis of RCD have considered this condition as a part of the broad spectrum of CCD and therefore provide an analysis of risk factors for developing complications of CD as a whole [22–25]. On the contrary, other papers have considered RCD as a definite clinical entity and provided data on outcome of RCD alone [26–32].

## Mortality in Complicated Coeliac Disease and Refractory Coeliac Disease

Since CCD is very rare (estimated annual incidence of 0.2% of all coeliac patients) [23], contemporary data for mortality in RCD and CCD remains scarce [22–32]. Table 1 provides an overview of the most relevant international studies addressing the issue of prognosis in RCD [22–32]. Some of these studies by large international referral centres have assessed long-term outcomes and mortality in series of RCD patients only [26–32]. Others, on the contrary, have reported data on more heterogeneous cohorts represented by CCD as a whole, rather than only RCD [22–25].

**Table 1** Studies evaluating natural history and mortality in complicated coeliac disease and refractory coeliac disease

| Study | Country | RCD Patients, n° | Evolution into EATL | Mortality | 5-Year survival |
|---|---|---|---|---|---|
| *Studies on RCD only* | | | | | |
| Malamut G, 2009 [26] | France | Total = 57 RCD1 = 14 RCD2 = 43 | Total = 18 (32%) RCD1 = 2 (14%) RCD2 = 16 (37%) | Total = 29 (51%) RCD1 = 3 (21%) RCD2 = 26 (60%) | RCD1 = 93% RCD2 = 44% |
| Al-Toma A, 2009 [27] | The Netherlands | Total = 93 RCD1 = 43 RCD2 = 50 | Total = 26 (28%) RCD1 = 0 RCD2 = 26 (52%) | Total = 54 (58%) RCD1 = 3 (7%) RCD2 = 28 (56%) RCD + EATL = 23 (88%) | RCD1 = 96% RCD2 = 58% RCD2 + EATL = 8% |
| Rubio-Tapia A, 2009 [28] | USA | Total = 57 RCD1 = 42 RCD2 = 15 | Total = 10 (17%) RCD1 = 0 RCD2 = 10 (67%) | Total = 15 (26%) RCD1 = 8 (19%) RCD2 = 7 (46%) | RCD1 = 80% RCD2 = 45% |
| Daum S, 2009 [29] | Germany | Total = 32 RCD1 = 23 RCD2 = 9 | Total = 4 (12%) RCD1 = 0 RCD2 = 4 (44%) | Total = 8 (25%) RCD1 = 4 (17%) RCD2 = 4 (44%) | RCD1 = 90% RCD2 = 53% |
| Roshan B, 2011 [30] | USA | Total = 29 RCD1 = 24 RCD2 = 5 | Total = 2 (7%) RCD1 = 0 RCD2 = 2 (40%) | Total = 2 (7%) RCD1 = 0 RCD2 = 2 (40%) | RCD1 = 100% RCD2 = 60% (2 years f-up) |
| Nasr I, 2014 [31] | United Kingdom | Total – 30 RCD1 = 0 RCD2 = 30 | None | None | All alive |
| Ilus T, 2014 [32] | Finland | Total = 44 RCD1 = 30 RCD2 = 10 [a]RCDx = 4 | Total = 4 (9%) RCD1 = 1 (3%) RCD2 = 3 (30%) RCDx = 0 | Total = 6 (14%) RCD1 = 3 (10%) RCD2 = 3 (30%) RCDx = 0 | NA |
| *Studies on complicated coeliac disease* | | | | | |
| Biagi, 2014 [22] | Multicenter European | Total = 71 RCD1 = 39 RCD2 = 32 | Total = 12 (17%) RCD1 = 1 (2%) RCD2 = 11 (40%) | Total = 13 (18%) RCD1 = 7 (18%) RCD2 = 6 (19%) | NA |

(continued)

**Table 1** (continued)

| Study | Country | RCD Patients, n° | Evolution into EATL | Mortality | 5-Year survival |
|-------|---------|------------------|---------------------|-----------|-----------------|
| Biagi, 2014 [23] | Italy | Total = 7<br>RCD1 = 5<br>RCD2 = 2 | NA | Total = 3 (43%)<br>RCD1 = 3 (60%)<br>RCD2 = 0 (0%) | NA |
| Biagi, 2014 [24] | Italy | Total = 30<br>RCD1 = 20<br>RCD2 = 3<br>ªRCDx = 7 | NA | Overall mortality CCD 43%, with no difference for each single subtypes | No difference within subtypes |
| Biagi, 2018 [25] | Italy | Total = 6<br>RCD1 = 6<br>RCD2 = 0 | None | Mortality rate for CCD 66 per 1000 person/years (95% CI 1–2.3) | NA |

*RCD1* refractory coeliac disease type1, *RCD2* refractory coeliac disease type 2, *EATL* enteropathy-associated T-cell lymphoma, *CCD* complicated coeliac disease, *n* number, *f-up* follow-up, *95% CI* 95% confidence interval
ªFor these patients it was not possible to discriminate between type 1 and type 2

# Predictors and Risk Factors for Complicated Coeliac Disease

In the last two decades it has emerged that the mortality of coeliac patients depends on several factors [reviewed in 3]. While strict adherence to a gluten free diet (GFD) is known to play a protective role for the onset of complications [5, 6], a classical clinical presentation of CD and advanced age at diagnosis were associated with increased mortality [6]. Other factors such as a long diagnostic delay and male sex were initially described as risk factors for complications [6, 33], but were not subsequently confirmed [22, 23]. Finally, HLA genotype was shown to correlate with clinical types of CD and onset of complications, with a higher risk of complications in DQ2 homozygous patients, i.e. those carrying a double dose of HLA-DQ2 molecules [34, 35]. Although these results allow the delineation of a specific phenotype of coeliac patients at increased risk of poor long-term prognosis, so far, due to the selection bias arising from all these patients being followed-up in referral centres, data on the prevalence and incidence of RCD and CCD in CD patients are still lacking. Only one single multicentre longitudinal study from Italy has calculated the risk of developing CCD [25]. In this study, 17 out of 2225 coeliac patients diagnosed over a 15-year period and followed-up for a median of 79 months (IQR 37–125) developed a complication (overall incidence of complications 11 per 10,000 persons/year, 95% CI 6–17 per 10,000 persons/year). The list of complications includes six type 1 RCD, 4 EATL, 5 SBC, 2 abdominal B-cell lymphomas. The key message of this study is that the risk of complications in CD is strictly related to the age at diagnosis of CD and clinical pattern of CD. More precisely, the risk of complications progressively increases as the age at diagnosis of CD increases. While the incidence of complications is very low in coeliac patients diagnosed before the age of 40 years (1/2000 persons/year), it is 1/1000 persons/year for those diagnosed between 41 and 60 years, and almost 1/100 persons/year for those diagnosed after the age of 60. In coeliac patients diagnosed after the age of 60 years, the risk of developing complications is 18 times higher than in patients diagnosed in the age group 18–40 years and nine times higher than in patients aged 41–60 years at diagnosis. The clinical type of CD is the other very important predictor of complications. Risk is virtually absent for asymptomatic patients. It is 1/2500 persons/year in non-classical CD, but rises to more than 1/400 persons/year in classical CD. The risk of developing complications is seven times higher in patients with a classical presentation than in those with a non-classical presentation, and increases exponentially comparing classical and non-classical patients to asymptomatic ones. Finally, the incidence of complications does not vary with the year of diagnosis, sex and centre where the diagnosis of CD was made.

As far as laboratory markers are concerned, another Italian multicentre study evaluating the natural history and prognosis of CCD found that coeliac patients who would later develop a complication had significantly lower haemoglobin, albumin and cholesterol together with increased levels of ESR and CRP than conventional uncomplicated coeliac patients [24]. Although in both these studies a specific risk analysis for each single subtype of complication was not performed [24, 25], data on clinical phenotypes of coeliac patients who developed a complication were very homogeneous regardless of the specific type of complication. Therefore, it can be assumed that these studies are entirely representative also of RCD. To date, there are no studies that have compared the risk of developing RCD with the risk of developing different types of complications. Only a recent Dutch study estimated the risk of developing EATL and SBC [36] and the results are comparable to the Italian studies [22–25], thus confirming that complications of CD can be grouped together.

## Prognostic Score for Complicated Coeliac Disease: The PROCONSUL SCORE

Currently, there is only one score available to estimate the risk of developing CCD in coeliac patients at time of diagnosis of CD [22]. This score was developed thanks to a large European observational multicentre case-control study evaluating 116 cases of CCD and 181 uncomplicated coeliac controls. This score is a three-level numeric score developed on the basis of a conditional logistic model including diagnostic delay and pattern of clinical presentation of CD as main prognostic factors. According to the PROCONSUL score risk of complications is low in patients presenting with non-classical/asymptomatic CD regardless of diagnostic delay. Patients presenting with classical symptoms and a long diagnostic delay (>6 months) have an intermediate risk. Finally, patients presenting with classical symptoms of malabsorption and short diagnostic delay (<6 months) are at high risk of developing CCD. Although this score represents a first attempt to optimise the follow-up of adult coeliac patients, it does not take into account age at diagnosis of CD, HLA typing and laboratory markers such as anaemia or hypoalbuminaemia. Considering that the majority of patients with CCD included in this study were affected by RCD (71 RCD out of 128 complications, 55%), we believe this score can be useful not only to evaluate the risk of developing CCD as a whole, but also to estimate the risk of RCD alone. Nevertheless, further prospective multicentre studies on larger cohorts are needed to build a specific prognostic score based on predictors already available at time of diagnosis of CD in order to assess the risk of developing RCD only.

## Predictors and Risk Factors for Poor Outcomes in Refractory Coeliac Disease

Once the diagnosis of RCD is confirmed and other causes of VA have been excluded [37], some elements need to be part of a thorough workout in order to estimate prognosis of these patients. They include the classification of RCD based on phenotypical assessment of aberrant IELs (RCD 1 vs. RCD 2), on the clinical modality of onset of refractoriness to a GFD (primary vs. secondary), and on the evaluation of full blood count and albumin levels.

### Clinical and Molecular Classification of Refractory Coeliac Disease

RCD can be classified either according to the phenotype of IELs (type 1 vs. type 2 RCD), or on the basis of a clinical criterion evaluating primary or secondary refractoriness to a GFD [17]. Although the distinction between type 1 and type 2 RCD based on the immunophenotype of IELs is the most widely adopted, both these ways of classifying RCD are relevant in terms of prognosis [17, 26–32].

As highlighted in Table 1, outcomes and mortality widely differ between type 1 and type 2 RCD. RCD 2 is associated with poor prognosis despite conventional therapeutic intervention, with a 5-year survival rate of 44–58% [17, 26–32]. The high mortality in RCD 2 is mainly due to the progression into overt EATL (up to 50% of RCD 2 evolves into EATL within 5 years from diagnosis) [17, 26–32]. The hallmark of type 2 RCD is a population of clonal aberrant IELs CD3$^-$, CD3epsilon$^+$, CD8$^-$, CD103$^+$, which can be detected also in EATL. So, some authors proposed the term pre-EATL to identify type 2 RCD [7]. On the contrary, this clonal population of IELs is absent in RCD 1. Therefore, response to treatment and prognosis in RCD 1 is significantly better than in RCD 2. However, although RCD1 presents a regular phenotype of IELs and evolution into EATL is almost anecdotal [17, 22, 26, 32], mortality rates in RCD 1 are nevertheless higher than in conventional uncomplicated CD [17, 27–32]. Continuous monitoring of aberrant IELs is mandatory in the follow-up of RCD patients and more accurate than single snapshot analysis for predicting evolution into EATL [38]. Therefore, it can be inferred that the classification of RCD based on the phenotypical assessment of IELs has an intrinsic prognostic value.

The second classification of RCD is based on a clinical criterion distinguishing between a primary and a secondary form of refractoriness to a strict GFD [10, 17, 24]. This classification can be attributed not only to RCD but in general to the modality of onset of any complication of CD and therefore is more indicative of the natural history of CCD. A recent Italian multicentre study investigating the natural history of 87 patients affected by a form of CCD, showed that this clinical classification has a relevant prognostic value. In this study, it was demonstrated that on the basis of the initial response to a GFD it is possible to identify two different clinical forms of CCD, characterized by substantial differences in terms of survival. A 49% 5-year survival rate was shown in patients in whom a GFD does not induce a significant remission of symptoms leading to the initial diagnosis of CD (primary refractoriness). On the contrary, a statistically different 75% 5-year survival rate emerged in patients in whom the complication of CD arose after an initial remission of symptoms (secondary refractoriness) [24]. Moreover, in patients with primary complications, anemia, hypoalbuminaemia and increased inflammatory markers were found more commonly than in those with secondary complications. It is interesting to note that EATL, UJI and SBC were more frequent among primary than in secondary cases. On the contrary, RCD 1 was more common in secondary cases. A possible explanation may be that in coeliac patients primarily unresponsive to a GFD, a malignant complication had already been triggered, thus confirming a more serious clinical picture.

As far as laboratory exams are concerned, low haemoglobin levels ($\leq$11 g/dL), hypoalbuminaemia ($\leq$3.2 g/dL) and low cholesterol levels are more common in patients with RCD 2, thus confirming a more severe clinical picture [17, 24, 26–28, 39]. More specifically, anaemia and hypoalbuminaemia are relevant predictors of poor outcomes in RCD [39], as discussed below.

## Scores to Predict Survival in Refractory Coeliac Disease

A few studies evaluated prognostic factors in RCD [17, 26, 28, 39]. Rubio-Tapia et al. developed two scores predicting outcomes in RCD [28, 39]. The first one is a clinical staging model based on the cumulative effect on survival of five prognostic factors evaluated at time of diagnosis of RCD [28]. They include albumin ($\leq$3.2 g/dL), haemoglobin ($\leq$11 g/dL), age ($\geq$65 years old), presence of aberrant IELs and severe histological damage (Marsh 3c). Each factor counted for one point and the final score is obtained by summing together all the points (each factor is one point; minimum 0, maximum 5). On the basis of the final score obtained, three prognostic categories are identified. Patients belonging to stage I (score 0–1) had a 5-year cumulative survival of 96% (95% CI 89%–100%), patients in stage II (score 2–3) had a 5-year cumulative survival of 71% (95% CI 47%–95%) and patients in stage III (score 4–5) had a very poor 5-year survival of 19% (95% CI 0%–41%). This staging system has the major advantage that the prognostic factors can be evaluated at time of diagnosis of RCD, but the main limitation of a single-centre experience with the potential of a referral bias [28].

A second score has been proposed more recently. This is a model to predict survival in RCD that has been developed thanks to data from a multinational registry [39]. The international cohort was composed of 232 patients diagnosed with RCD in seven centres. By means of a Cox proportional hazard regression a three-factor risk score was created to estimate 5-year survival. The three prognostic factors included in the model are age at diagnosis of RCD >40 years (per 20-year increase HR 2.21, 95% CI 1.38–3.55), abnormal IELs (HR 2.85; 95% CI 1.22–6.62), and albumin (per 0.5 unit increase, HR 0.72; 95% CI 0.61–0.85). Modalities of score computation and correlation with 5-year survival are summarised in Tables 2 and 3.

**Table 2** Three-factor risk score (derived from Rubio-Tapia et al. [39]) system

| Predictor | Value | Points |
|---|---|---|
| Abnormal IELs | Yes | 3 |
| | No | 0 |
| Albumin (g/dL) | >4.5 | 0 |
| | 4.0–4.50 | 1 |
| | 3.5–3.99 | 2 |
| | 3.0–3.49 | 3 |
| | 2.5–2.99 | 4 |
| | 2.0–2.49 | 5 |
| | 1.5–1.99 | 6 |
| | < 1.5 | 7 |
| Age at diagnosis of RCD (years) | 0–39 | 0 |
| | 40–59 | 2 |
| | 60–79 | 4 |
| | > 80 | 6 |

*IELs* intraepithelial lymphocytes, *RCD* refractory coeliac disease

**Table 3** Reletionship between the result of the three-factor risk score shown in table 2 and 5-year survival in refractory coeliac disease (derived from Rubio-Tapia et al. [39])

| Quartile | Score result | 5-Years survival (95% CI) |
|---|---|---|
| I | 0–4 | 97.6% (62.2–99.7) |
| II | 5–7 | 83.2% (66.1–92.0) |
| III | 8 or 9 | 60.5% (39.9–74.3) |
| IV | ≥10 | 48.5% (33.3–61.7) |

*95% CI* 95% confidence interval

The main advantage of this score is the use of predictors commonly available in clinical practice.

## Conclusions

Contemporary data on outcomes in RCD still indicate a low rate of response to therapies and a high mortality, particularly in type 2 RCD. Identification of the phenotype of coeliac patients at higher risk of developing complications and strict follow-up are mandatory in order to try to prevent poor outcomes. This includes patients presenting with severe malabsorption, advanced age at diagnosis of CD and primary refractoriness to a strict GFD. Once diagnosis of RCD is confirmed, distinction between type 1 and type 2, together with a thorough biochemical, endoscopic and radiological workout is necessary to identify patients at higher risk of a poor outcome, who may require more aggressive and targeted therapies.

## References

1. Lebwohl B, Sanders DS, Green PHR. Coeliac disease. Lancet. 2018;391:70–81.
2. Singh P, Arora A, Strand TA, et al. Global prevalence of celiac disease: systematic review and meta-analysis. Clin Gastroenterol Hepatol. 2018;16:823–36.
3. Biagi F, Corazza GR. Mortality in celiac disease. Nat Rev Gastroenterol Hepatol. 2010;7:158–62.
4. West J. Celiac disease and its complications: a time traveller's perspective. Gastroenterology. 2009;136:32–4.
5. Holmes GK, Prior P, Lane MR, Pope D, Allan RN. Malignancy in coeliac disease--effect of a gluten free diet. Gut. 1989;30:333–8.
6. Corrao G, Corazza GR, Bagnardi V, Brusco G, Ciacci C, Cottone M, et al. Mortality in patients with coeliac disease and their relatives: a cohort study. Lancet. 2001;358:356–61.
7. Cellier C, Delabesse E, Helmer C, Patey N, Matuchansky C, Jabri B, et al. Refractory sprue, coeliac disease, and enteropathy-associated T-cell lymphoma. French Coeliac Disease Study Group. Lancet. 2000;356:203–8.
8. Brousse N, Meijer JW. Malignant complications of coeliac disease. Best Pract Res Clin Gastroenterol. 2005;19:401–12.
9. Ludvigsson JF. Mortality and malignancy in celiac disease. Gastrointest Endosc Clin N Am. 2012;22:705–22.
10. Malamut G, Cellier C. Complications of coeliac disease. Best Pract Res Clin Gastroenterol. 2015;29:451–8.
11. Stenson WF, Newberry R, Lorenz R, Baldus C, Civitelli R. Increased prevalence of celiac disease and need for routine screening among patients with osteoporosis. Arch Intern Med. 2005;165:393–9.
12. Corazza GR, Di Sario A, Cecchetti L, Tarozzi C, Corrao G, Bernardi M, et al. Bone mass and metabolism in patients with celiac disease. Gastroenterology. 1995;109:122–8.
13. Efthymakis K, Milano A, Laterza F, Serio M, Neri M. Iron deficiency anemia despite effective gluten-free diet in celiac disease: diagnostic role of small bowel capsule endoscopy. Dig Liver Dis. 2017;49:412–6.

14. Cosnes J, Cellier C, Viola S, Colombel JF, Michaud L, Sarles J, et al. Incidence of autoimmune diseases in celiac disease: protective effect of the gluten-free diet. Clin Gastroenterol Hepatol. 2008;6:753–8.

15. Collin P, Reunala T, Pukkala E, Laippala P, Keyriläinen O, Pasternack A. Coeliac disease--associated disorders and survival. Gut. 1994;35:1215–8.

16. Schiepatti A, Sprio E, Sanders DS, Lovati E, Biagi F. Coeliac disease and obstetric and gynaecological disorders: where are we now? Eur J Gastroenterol Hepatol. 2019;31:425–33.

17. Rubio-Tapia A, Murray JA. Classification and management of refractory coeliac disease. Gut. 2010;59:547–57.

18. Biagi F, Lorenzini P, Corazza GR. Literature review on the clinical relationship between ulcerative jejunoileitis, coeliac disease, and enteropathy-associated T-cell. Scand J Gastroenterol. 2000;35:785–90.

19. Di Sabatino A, Biagi F, Gobbi PG, Corazza GR. How I treat enteropathy-associated T-cell lymphoma. Blood. 2012;119:2458–68.

20. Leslie LA, Lebwohl B, Neugut AI, Gregory Mears J, Bhagat G, Green PH. Incidence of lymphoproliferative disorders in patients with celiac disease. Am J Hematol. 2012;87:754–9.

21. Raghav K, Overman MJ. Small bowel adenocarcinomas--existing evidence and evolving paradigms. Nat Rev Clin Oncol. 2013;10:534–44.

22. Biagi F, Schiepatti A, Malamut G, Marchese A, Cellier C, Bakker SF, et al. PROgnosticating COeliac patieNts SUrvivaL: the PROCONSUL score. PLoS One. 2014;9:e84163.

23. Biagi F, Gobbi P, Marchese A, Borsotti E, Zingone F, Ciacci C, et al. Low incidence but poor prognosis of complicated coeliac disease: a retrospective multicentre study. Dig Liver Dis. 2014;46:227–30.

24. Biagi F, Marchese A, Ferretti F, Ciccocioppo R, Schiepatti A, Volta U, et al. A multicentre case control study on complicated coeliac disease: two different patterns of natural history, two different prognoses. BMC Gastroenterol. 2014;14:139.

25. Biagi F, Schiepatti A, Maiorano G, Fraternale G, Agazzi S, Zingone F, et al. Risk of complications in coeliac patients depends on age at diagnosis and type of clinical presentation. Dig Liver Dis. 2018;50:549–52.

26. Malamut G, Afchain P, Verkarre V, Lecomte T, Amiot A, Damotte D, et al. Presentation and long-term follow-up of refractory celiac disease: comparison of type I with type II. Gastroenterology. 2009;136:81–90.

27. Al-Toma A, Verbeek WH, Hadithi M, von Blomberg BM, Mulder CJ. Survival in refractory coeliac disease and enteropathy-associated T-cell lymphoma: retrospective evaluation of single-centre experience. Gut. 2007;56:1373–8.

28. Rubio-Tapia A, Kelly DG, Lahr BD, Dogan A, Wu TT, Murray JA. Clinical staging and survival in refractory celiac disease: a single center experience. Gastroenterology. 2009;136:99–107.

29. Daum S, Ipczynski R, Schumann M, Wahnschaffe U, Zeitz M, Ullrich R. High rates of complications and substantial mortality in both types of refractory sprue. Eur J Gastroenterol Hepatol. 2009;21:66–70.

30. Roshan B, Leffler DA, Jamma S, Dennis M, Sheth S, Falchuk K, et al. The incidence and clinical spectrum of refractory celiac disease in a North American referral center. Am J Gastroenterol. 2011;106:923–8.

31. Nasr I, Nasr I, Beyers C, Chang F, Donnelly S, Ciclitira PJ. Recognising and managing refractory coeliac disease: a tertiary centre experience. Nutrients. 2015;7:9896–907.

32. Ilus T, Kaukinen K, Virta LJ, Huhtala H, Mäki M, Kurppa K, et al. Refractory coeliac disease in a country with a high prevalence of clinically-diagnosed coeliac disease. Aliment Pharmacol Ther. 2014;39:418–25.

33. Leffler DA, Dennis M, Hyett B, Kelly E, Schuppan D, Kelly CP. Etiologies and predictors of diagnosis in nonresponsive celiac disease. Clin Gastroenterol Hepatol. 2007;5:445–50.

34. Al-Toma A, Goerres MS, Meijer JW, Peña AS, Crusius JB, Mulder CJ. Human leukocyte antigen-DQ2 homozygosity and the development of refractory celiac disease and enteropathy-associated T-cell lymphoma. Clin Gastroenterol Hepatol. 2006;4:315–9.

35. Biagi F, Bianchi PI, Vattiato C, Marchese A, Trotta L, Badulli C, et al. Influence of HLA-DQ2 and DQ8 on severity in celiac disease. J Clin Gastroenterol. 2012;46:46–50.
36. van Gils T, Nijeboer P, Overbeek LI, Hauptmann M, Castelijn DA, Bouma G, et al. Risks for lymphoma and gastrointestinal carcinoma in patients with newly diagnosed adult-onset celiac disease: consequences for follow-up: celiac disease, lymphoma and GI carcinoma. United European Gastroenterol J. 2018;6:1485–95.
37. Schiepatti A, Sanders DS, Zuffada M, Luinetti O, Iraqi A, Biagi F. Overview in the clinical management of patients with seronegative villous atrophy. Eur J Gastroenterol Hepatol. 2019;31:409–17.
38. Liu H, Brais R, Lavergne-Slove A, Jeng Q, Payne K, Ye H, et al. Continual monitoring of intraepithelial lymphocyte immunophenotype and clonality is more important than snapshot analysis in the surveillance of refractory coeliac disease. Gut. 2010;59:452–60.
39. Rubio-Tapia A, Malamut G, Verbeek WH, van Wanrooij RL, Leffler DA, Niveloni SI, et al. Creation of a model to predict survival in patients with refractory coeliac disease using a multinational registry. Aliment Pharmacol Ther. 2016;44:704–14.

# Enteropathy-Associated T-Cell Lymphoma

**David Sibon and Olivier Hermine**

## Definition

Enteropathy-associated T-cell lymphoma (EATL) is a neoplasm of intraepithelial T cells that occurs in individuals with celiac disease (CD) [1].

## Epidemiology

EATL is a rare lymphoma that typically occurs in the sixth and seventh decades of life, with a slight male predominance. It is more frequent in areas with a high prevalence of CD.

In the French Lymphopath Network study, there were 15 new cases of EATL diagnosed per year in France, among the 8000 new cases of non-cutaneous lymphomas that were reviewed [2]. In a case-control study from the Dutch nationwide population-based pathology database, the risk of T-cell lymphoma, predominantly EATL, was strongly associated with CD diagnosis (RR = 35.8) [3]. The highest absolute risk of 4.3% for T-cell lymphoma was reported in males between the ages 50 and 80 years when CD was diagnosed at age 50 years. CD and EATL were simultaneously diagnosed in 50% of the patients.

D. Sibon (✉) · O. Hermine
Hematology Department, Necker University Hospital, Assistance Publique – Hôpitaux de Paris, Paris, France

Université de Paris, Paris, France

French NCI-labeled network of Centers of Expertise for Lymphomas Associated with Celiac disease (CELAC), Paris, France
e-mail: david.sibon@aphp.fr

© Springer Nature Switzerland AG 2022
G. Malamut, N. Cerf-Bensussan (eds.), *Refractory Celiac Disease*,
https://doi.org/10.1007/978-3-030-90142-4_11

EATL is associated with the HLA-DQA1*05:01 and HLA-DQB1*02:01 genotypes [4]. More than 90% of EATL patients carry HLA-DQ2.5 heterodimers encoded by HLA-DQA1*05 and HLA-DQB1*02 alleles, either in cis or trans configuration [5]. The main risk factors of developing EATL are the presence of refractory CD type II (RCD-II), non-observance of a strict gluten-free diet, homozygosity for the HLA-DQ2 allele, and age.

## Pathology and Genetics

Macroscopically, EATL may form ulcerating nodules, plaques, strictures or an exophytic mass. The mesenteric lymph nodes are commonly involved, sometimes in the absence of macroscopic evidence of intestinal infiltration. Microscopically, the neoplastic lymphocytes exhibit a wide range of cytological aspects. Most EATL show pleomorphic medium-sized to large cells. Some cases exhibit predominant large cell or anaplastic morphology [1]. Angiocentricity, angioinvasion and necrosis are frequently observed. Most EATL have an admixture of inflammatory cells, including large numbers of histiocytes and eosinophils. The intestinal mucosa adjacent to EATL usually shows features of CD (villous atrophy, crypt hyperplasia, and intraepithelial lymphocytosis). The neoplastic lymphocytes are usually CD3+/− CD5− CD7+ CD4− CD8− CD30+ CD103+ cytotoxicity+ (perforin, granzyme B, TIA-1). Most EATL either displays gains of the 9q34 region, or alternatively shows deletions of 16q12.1. Gains of chromosomes 1q and 5q are frequent. EATL displays a complex mutational profile dominated by highly recurrent gain-of-functions mutations of JAK1 and STAT3, frequently associated with mutations which activate the NF-κB pathway [6]. TCR genes are clonally rearranged in virtually all EATL.

## Clinical Features

EATL occurs most commonly (>90%) in the jejunum or proximal ileum. Multifocal lesions are observed in about half of the cases. Stomach and colon are other common gastro-intestinal sites. Extra digestive sites are occasionally involved (lymph nodes, spleen, skin, brain).

The most common presenting symptoms are abdominal pain (80–90%) and weight loss (50–80%) [7–9]. Patients present with intestinal perforation or obstruction, each in 20–40% of cases. Intra-abdominal lymph nodes are observed in 20–35%, and other sites in 5–10% (mediastinal lymph nodes, bone marrow, lung, liver, skin, brain).

# Staging

CT-scan and PET-scan are used for staging EATL. Upper endoscopy may be useful for assessing the uninvolved mucosa, especially for detecting RCD-II.

# Prognosis

The prognosis of EATL is poor, with a five-year overall survival (OS) of 10–15% [10, 11]. The international prognostic index (IPI) and the prognostic index for peripheral T-cell lymphoma (PTCL), unspecified (PIT) have limited predictive value for outcome of EATL. In 2015, an EATL prognostic index (EPI) was constructed, based on the presence of B-symptom (defined as the presence of fever and/or night sweats, excluding weight loss), and IPI score [11]. Three risk groups were distinguished: A high-risk group, characterized by the presence of B-symptoms [median OS of two months]; an intermediate-risk group, comprising patients without B-symptoms and an IPI score ≥2 (7 months); and a low-risk group, representing patients without B-symptoms and an IPI score of 0 to 1 (34 months).

# Treatment

With surgery alone, no patient is alive at five years, whereas with chemotherapy, some patients may expect long-term survival [7–9].

In the retrospective study from the International Peripheral T-Cell Lymphoma Project, the use of anthracycline-containing chemotherapy improved the OS and failure-free survival (FFS) compared with other therapies or no therapy [8]. In this report, none of the patients received consolidative high-dose therapy/autologous stem-cell transplantation (HDT/ASCT) in first remission. The five-year OS was 20%, and the five-year FFS was only 4%.

In a French retrospective study on 37 EATL patients, serum albumin level >21.6 g/L, chemotherapy and reductive surgery were all significantly associated with increased OS [9].

The Scotland and Newcastle Lymphoma Group (SNLG) evaluated in a population-based study the chemotherapy regimen IVE/MTX (ifosfamide, etoposide, epirubicin/methotrexate) followed by HDT/ASCT in 26 patients aged 36–69 years [7]. Fourteen patients underwent HDT/ASCT. For the 26 patients, five-year progression-free survival (PFS) and OS were 52% and 60%, respectively. These favourable results encouraged to prospectively assess the feasibility of this approach in a multi-centre UK phase 2 study for aggressive T-cell lymphoma [12]. Unfortunately, target recruitment was not reached, with 21 PTCL, eight of which were EATL. After a median follow-up of 27 months, four EATL patients were alive and lymphoma-free, two had relapsed from CR and two had died during IVE-MTX.

The phase 2 study of the Nordic Lymphoma Group (NLG-T-01) included 21 EATL patients [13]. An induction regimen of six cycles of biweekly CHOEP (cyclophosphamide, doxorubicin, vincristine, etoposide, and prednisone) was administered (in patients age > 60 years, etoposide was omitted). Patients in complete or partial remission proceeded to consolidation with HDT/ASCT. The five-year PFS and OS for the 21 EATL patients were 38% and 48%, respectively.

The European Group for Blood and Marrow Transplantation (EBMT) retrospectively evaluated HDT/ASCT as a consolidation or salvage strategy for 44 EATL patients aged 35–72 years, between 2000 and 2010 [14]. Thirty-one patients (70%) were in first complete or partial remission at the time of the HDT/ASCT. With a median follow-up of 46 months, four-year PFS and OS were 54% and 59%, respectively.

In the prospective study from the T Cell Project, the three-year PFS and OS of 65 EATL patients were 28% and 30%, respectively [15]. In this study, all patients had anthracycline-based regimens, and only three had HDT/ASCT in first remission.

In summary, based on non-randomized studies, the following conclusions may be drawn:

- Surgery may be considered in first place but never alone
- A chemotherapy-based treatment should be considered whenever feasible
- The use of anthracycline-containing regimen seems to improve the FFS and OS
- After cyclophosphamide, doxorubicine, vincristine, prednisone (CHOP) without consolidative HDT-ASCT, five-year OS is only 10–20%
- Both prospective phase 2 studies (UK and NLG-T-01) shared common drugs during induction regimen: alkylating agent, anthracycline, vincristine, etoposide and prednisone. These drugs could be used as backbone for future prospective trials.
- HDT/ASCT is feasible in EATL patients ≤70 years and may induce long-term survival, however, approximately half of the patients with a planned HDT-ASCT are actually transplanted.

## Conclusion and Perspective

EATL is a rare lymphoma with a poor prognosis. It is an unmet medical needs for which new therapies are eagerly awaited. Very few clinical trials include EATL, and in almost all of these trials, EATL are mixed with other more common PTCL, making it difficult to properly assess new treatments in EATL patients. To the best of our knowledge, only one clinical trial specifically dedicated to EATL is ongoing: this phase 2 study is evaluating Brentuximab Vedotin associated with cyclophosphamide, doxorubicine, and prednisone (CHP) followed by consolidation with HDT/ASCT as frontline treatment of patients with EATL (ClinicalTrials.gov Identifier: NCT03217643).

# References

1. Swerdlow SH, Campo E, Harris NL, Jaffe ES, Pileri S, Stein H, et al. WHO classification of tumors of haematopoietic and lymphoid tissues (revised 4th edition). Lyon, France: IARC; 2017.
2. Laurent C, Baron M, Amara N, Haioun C, Dandoit M, Maynadié M, et al. Impact of expert pathologic review of lymphoma diagnosis: study of patients from the French Lymphopath network. J Clin Oncol. 2017;35(18):2008–17.
3. van Gils T, Nijeboer P, Overbeek LI, Hauptmann M, Castelijn DA, Bouma G, et al. Risks for lymphoma and gastrointestinal carcinoma in patients with newly diagnosed adult-onset celiac disease: consequences for follow-up: celiac disease, lymphoma and GI carcinoma. United Eur Gastroenterol J. 2018;6(10):1485–95.
4. Al-Toma A, Goerres MS, Meijer JWR, Peña AS, Crusius JBA, Mulder CJJ. Human leukocyte antigen-DQ2 homozygosity and the development of refractory celiac disease and enteropathy-associated T-cell lymphoma. Clin Gastroenterol Hepatol. 2006;4(3):315–9.
5. Howell WM, Leung ST, Jones DB, Nakshabendi I, Hall MA, Lanchbury JS, et al. HLA-DRB, -DQA, and -DQB polymorphism in celiac disease and enteropathy-associated T-cell lymphoma. Common features and additional risk factors for malignancy. Hum Immunol. 1995;43(1):29–37.
6. Cording S, Lhermitte L, Malamut G, et al. Oncogenetic landscape of lymphomagenesis in coeliac disease. Gut. Published Online First: 2021. https://doi.org/10.1136/gutjnl-2020-322935.
7. Sieniawski M, Angamuthu N, Boyd K, Chasty R, Davies J, Forsyth P, et al. Evaluation of enteropathy-associated T-cell lymphoma comparing standard therapies with a novel regimen including autologous stem cell transplantation. Blood. 2010;115(18):3664–70.
8. Delabie J, Holte H, Vose JM, Ullrich F, Jaffe ES, Savage KJ, et al. Enteropathy-associated T-cell lymphoma: clinical and histological findings from the international peripheral T-cell lymphoma project. Blood. 2011;118(1):148–55.
9. Malamut G, Chandesris O, Verkarre V, Meresse B, Callens C, Macintyre E, et al. Enteropathy associated T cell lymphoma in celiac disease: a large retrospective study. Dig Liver Dis. 2013;45(5):377–84.
10. Nijeboer P, de Baaij LR, Visser O, Witte BI, Cillessen SAGM, Mulder CJ, et al. Treatment response in enteropathy associated T-cell lymphoma; survival in a large multicenter cohort. Am J Hematol. 2015;90(6):493 8.
11. de Baaij LR, Berkhof J, van de Water JMW, Sieniawski MK, Radersma M, Verbeek WHM, et al. A new and validated clinical prognostic model (EPI) for Enteropathy-associated T-cell lymphoma. Clin Cancer Res. 2015;21(13):3013–9.
12. Phillips EH, Lannon MM, Lopes A, Chadwick H, Jones G, Sieniawski M, et al. High-dose chemotherapy and autologous stem cell transplantation in enteropathy-associated and other aggressive T-cell lymphomas: a UK NCRI/Cancer Research UK phase II study. Bone Marrow Transplant. 2019;54(3):465–8.
13. d'Amore F, Relander T, Lauritzsen GF, Jantunen E, Hagberg H, Anderson H, et al. Up-front autologous stem-cell transplantation in peripheral T-cell lymphoma: NLG-T-01. J Clin Oncol. 2012;30(25):3093–9.
14. Jantunen E, Boumendil A, Finel H, Luan J-J, Johnson P, Rambaldi A, et al. Autologous stem cell transplantation for enteropathy-associated T-cell lymphoma: a retrospective study by the EBMT. Blood. 2013;121(13):2529–32.
15. Foss FM, Horwitz SM, Civallero M, Bellei M, Marcheselli L, Kim WS, et al. Incidence and outcomes of rare T cell lymphomas from the T cell project: hepatosplenic, enteropathy associated and peripheral gamma delta T cell lymphomas. Am J Hematol. 2020;95(2):151–5.

Printed in the United States
by Baker & Taylor Publisher Services